T0263808

INTERVENTIONAL CARDIOLOGY CLINICS

www.interventional.theclinics.com

Editor-in-Chief

MATTHEW J. PRICE

Key Trials of the Decade

October 2020 • Volume 9 • Number 4

ELSEVIER

1600 John F. Kennedy Boulevard • Suite 1800 • Philadelphia, Pennsylvania, 19103-2899

http://www.theclinics.com

INTERVENTIONAL CARDIOLOGY CLINICS Volume 9, Number 4
October 2020 ISSN 2211-7458, ISBN-13: 978-0-323-77674-5

Editor: Joanna Collett
Developmental Editor: Donald Mumford

© **2020 Elsevier Inc. All rights reserved.**

This periodical and the individual contributions contained in it are protected under copyright by Elsevier, and the following terms and conditions apply to their use:

Photocopying
Single photocopies of single articles may be made for personal use as allowed by national copyright laws. Permission of the Publisher and payment of a fee is required for all other photocopying, including multiple or systematic copying, copying for advertising or promotional purposes, resale, and all forms of document delivery. Special rates are available for educational institutions that wish to make photocopies for non-profit educational classroom use. For information on how to seek permission visit www.elsevier.com/permissions or call: (+44) 1865 843830 (UK)/(+1) 215 239 3804 (USA).

Derivative Works
Subscribers may reproduce tables of contents or prepare lists of articles including abstracts for internal circulation within their institutions. Permission of the Publisher is required for resale or distribution outside the institution. Permission of the Publisher is required for all other derivative works, including compilations and translations (please consult www.elsevier.com/permissions).

Electronic Storage or Usage
Permission of the Publisher is required to store or use electronically any material contained in this periodical, including any article or part of an article (please consult www.elsevier.com/permissions). Except as outlined above, no part of this publication may be reproduced, stored in a retrieval system or transmitted in any form or by any means, electronic, mechanical, photocopying, recording or otherwise, without prior written permission of the Publisher.

Notice
No responsibility is assumed by the Publisher for any injury and/or damage to persons or property as a matter of products liability, negligence or otherwise, or from any use or operation of any methods, products, instructions or ideas contained in the material herein. Because of rapid advances in the medical sciences, in particular, independent verification of diagnoses and drug dosages should be made.

Although all advertising material is expected to conform to ethical (medical) standards, inclusion in this publication does not constitute a guarantee or endorsement of the quality or value of such product or of the claims made of it by its manufacturer.

Interventional Cardiology Clinics (ISSN 2211-7458) is published quarterly by Elsevier Inc., 360 Park Avenue South, New York, NY 10010-1710. Months of issue are January, April, July, and October. Subscription prices are USD 209 per year for US individuals, USD 495 for US institutions, USD 100 per year for US students, USD 209 per year for Canadian individuals, USD 590 for Canadian institutions, USD 100 per year for Canadian students, USD 296 per year for international individuals, USD 590 for international institutions, and USD 150 per year for international students. To receive student/resident rate, orders must be accompanied by name of affiliated institution, date of term, and the *signature* of program/residency coordinator on institution letterhead. Orders will be billed at individual rate until proof of status is received. Foreign air speed delivery is included in all *Clinics* subscription prices. All prices are subject to change without notice. **POSTMASTER:** Send address changes to *Interventional Cardiology Clinics*, Elsevier Health Sciences Division, Subscription Customer Service, 3251 Riverport Lane, Maryland Heights, MO 63043. **Customer Service: Telephone: 1-800-654-2452** (U.S. and Canada); **1-314-447-8871** (outside U.S. and Canada). **Fax: 1-314-447-8029. E-mail: journalscustomerservice-usa@elsevier.com (for print support); journalsonlinesupport-usa@elsevier.com (for online support).**

Reprints. For copies of 100 or more of articles in this publication, please contact the Commercial Reprints Department, Elsevier Inc., 360 Park Avenue South, New York, NY 10010-1710. Tel.: 212-633-3874; Fax: 212-633-3820; E-mail: reprints@elsevier.com.

CONTRIBUTORS

EDITOR-IN-CHIEF

MATTHEW J. PRICE, MD
Director, Cardiac Catheterization Laboratory,
Division of Cardiovascular Diseases, Scripps
Clinic, La Jolla, California, USA

AUTHORS

RASHA K. AL-LAMEE, MA, MB BS, MRCP, PhD
Interventional Cardiology Consultant and
Clinical Senior Lecturer, Imperial College
Healthcare NHS Trust, Imperial College
London, Hammersmith Hospital, London,
United Kingdom

ZAIN UL ABIDEEN ASAD, MD
Assistant Professor of Medicine,
Cardiovascular Disease Section, Department
of Medicine, University of Oklahoma Health
Sciences Center, Oklahoma City, Oklahoma,
USA

LORENZO AZZALINI, MD, PhD, MSc
The Zena and Michael A. Wiener
Cardiovascular Institute, Icahn School of
Medicine at Mount Sinai, New York, New
York, USA

USMAN BABER, MD, MS
Associate Professor of Medicine,
Cardiovascular Disease Section, Department
of Medicine, University of Oklahoma Health
Sciences Center, Oklahoma City, Oklahoma,
USA

MATTHIAS BOSSARD, MD
Cardiology Division, Heart Center, Luzerner
Kantonsspital, Luzern, Switzerland

WILLIAM F. FEARON, MD
Professor of Medicine (Cardiovascular
Medicine), Director of Interventional
Cardiology, Division of Cardiovascular
Medicine, Stanford Cardiovascular
Institute, Stanford University School
of Medicine, Stanford, California,
USA

DAVID P. LEE, MD
Associate Professor of Medicine
(Cardiovascular), Stanford University
Interventional Cardiology, Stanford,
California, USA

DAVID SCOTT LIM, MD
Divisions of Cardiovascular Medicine and
Pediatric Cardiology, Professor, Departments
of Medicine and Pediatrics, Medical Director,
Advanced Cardiac Valve Center, University of
Virginia, Charlottesville, Virginia, USA

RYAN MARKHAM, MBBS, FRACP
Stanford Hospital, Palo Alto, California,
USA; Department of Cardiovascular
Medicine, Stanford Hospital, Stanford,
California, USA

SHAMIR R. MEHTA, MD, MSc, FRCPC, FACC, FESC
Population Health Research Institute,
Professor of Medicine, McMaster University,
Hamilton General Hospital, Hamilton Health
Sciences, Hamilton, Ontario, Canada

RUSHI V. PARIKH, MD
Assistant Clinical Professor of Medicine,
Division of Cardiology, University of California,
Los Angeles, David Geffen School of
Medicine, Los Angeles, California, USA

MATTHEW J. PRICE, MD
Director, Cardiac Catheterization Laboratory,
Division of Cardiovascular Diseases, Scripps
Clinic, La Jolla, California, USA

RAHUL SHARMA, MBBS, FRACP
Stanford Hospital, Palo Alto, California,
USA; Director of Structural Interventions,
Department of Cardiovascular Medicine,
Stanford Hospital, Stanford, California,
USA

NISHTHA SODHI, MD, FACC, FASE
Assistant Professor, Structural and
Interventional Cardiology, Division of
Cardiovascular Medicine, Department of
Medicine, Advanced Cardiac Valve Center,

University of Virginia, Charlottesville, Virginia,
USA

GREGG W. STONE, MD
The Zena and Michael A. Wiener
Cardiovascular Institute, Icahn School of
Medicine at Mount Sinai, The Cardiovascular
Research Foundation, New York, New York,
USA

ZHI TEOH, MA, MBBChir, MRCP
Interventional Cardiology Fellow, Barts Health
NHS Trust, London, United Kingdom

CONTENTS

The "Achilles heel" of invasive coronary angiography is its inability to accurately localize which stenoses induce ischemia and warrant treatment. Fractional flow reserve (FFR) is a coronary wire-based physiologic index that measures the functional significance of epicardial stenoses, thereby overcoming this limitation. Over the past decade, the landmark FAME (Fractional Flow Reserve vs Angiography for Multivessel Evaluation) trials demonstrated the clinical utility of an FFR-guided strategy for percutaneous coronary intervention (PCI) compared with angiography-only PCI or medical therapy alone in patients with predominantly stable ischemic heart disease. These trials have spurred the current era of coronary-physiology–guided revascularization.

Although coronary artery bypass graft (CABG) surgery traditionally has been considered the gold standard for left main revascularization, percutaneous coronary intervention has evolved in the past decades so that it now represents a valid alternative to CABG in a large proportion of cases. The landmark Evaluation of XIENCE versus Coronary Artery Bypass Surgery for Effectiveness of Left Main Revascularization (EXCEL) trial is the largest contemporary randomized comparison assessing the impact of revascularization strategies for left main disease. This review discusses the background, rationale, design, results, and implications of the EXCEL trial.

Many patients presenting with ST-segment elevation myocardial infarction (STEMI) have multivessel coronary artery disease (CAD). Following successful primary percutaneous coronary intervention (PCI) of culprit lesion, whether to routinely revascularize nonculprit lesions or treat them medically has been debated. Recently, the large-scale, multinational COMPLETE trial definitively established benefit of routine, staged, angiographically guided nonculprit lesion PCI in reducing hard clinical outcomes, including the composite of death from cardiovascular causes or new myocardial infarction, with no major safety concerns. A strategy of complete revascularization with routine nonculprit lesion PCI in suitable lesions should be standard of care in STEMI with multivessel CAD.

KEY TRIALS OF THE DECADE

RELATED SERIES

Cardiology Clinics
Cardiac Electrophysiology Clinics
Heart Failure Clinics

THE CLINICS ARE NOW AVAILABLE ONLINE!

Access your subscription at:
www.theclinics.com

Physiology over Angiography to Determine Lesion Severity: the FAME Trials

Rushi V. Parikh, MD[a], William F. Fearon, MD[b],*

KEYWORDS

• Fractional flow reserve • FAME • Coronary physiology • Percutaneous coronary intervention

KEY POINTS

• Invasive coronary angiography is limited by the inability to accurately discriminate which stenoses produce ischemia and warrant revascularization; fractional flow reserve (FFR) overcomes this limitation by localizing and quantifying the ischemic potential of epicardial stenoses.

• The seminal Fractional Flow Reserve versus Angiography for Multivessel Evaluation (FAME) trial showed that FFR-guided percutaneous coronary intervention (PCI) significantly reduced the 1-year composite outcome of death, myocardial infarction (MI), or repeat revascularization compared with PCI guided by angiography alone in predominantly stable ischemic heart disease (SIHD) patients with multivessel disease.

• FAME 2 subsequently demonstrated that an FFR-based approach to PCI significantly improved the composite outcome of death, MI, or urgent revascularization compared with OMT in patients with SIHD; this difference was primarily driven by a substantial reduction in urgent revascularization.

• FFR-guided revascularization is currently recommended by the major societal guidelines for SIHD and is advocated for by the appropriate use criteria for both SIHD and acute coronary syndrome (nonculprit stenoses).

INTRODUCTION

Atherosclerotic coronary artery stenoses that induce substantial myocardial ischemia are the primary cause of angina pectoris and lead to adverse clinical outcomes.[1,2] Targeted revascularization of these ischemia-producing stenoses results in reduced angina and improved clinical outcomes.[3,4] Conversely, stenoses that fail to induce significant ischemia can be safely and effectively treated with medical therapy alone.[5,6]

Invasive coronary angiography is the gold-standard method for identifying coronary stenoses. However, the "Achilles heel" of angiography remains its inability to accurately distinguish which stenoses cause ischemia and warrant revascularization, particularly those in the intermediate range.[7,8] Noninvasive stress imaging modalities are similarly limited in their ability to identify ischemia-producing stenoses.[9] Fractional flow reserve (FFR), a coronary wire-based index that measures the physiologic (ie, functional) significance of epicardial coronary stenoses, overcomes these diagnostic limitations and accurately determines the ischemic potential of a given stenosis.[10] Over the past decade, the landmark Fractional Flow Reserve versus Angiography for Multivessel Evaluation (FAME) trials have established the clinical benefit of an FFR-directed strategy for percutaneous coronary intervention (PCI) and ushered in the contemporary era of invasive coronary

[a] Division of Cardiology, University of California, Los Angeles, David Geffen School of Medicine, 100 Medical Plaza, Suite 630 West, Los Angeles, CA 90095, USA; [b] Division of Cardiovascular Medicine, Stanford Cardiovascular Institute, Stanford University School of Medicine, 300 Pasteur Drive, Room H2103, Stanford, CA 94035, USA
* Corresponding author.
E-mail address: wfearon@stanford.edu
Twitter: @rushiparikh11 (R.V.P.); @wfearonmd (W.F.F.)

Intervent Cardiol Clin 9 (2020) 409–418
https://doi.org/10.1016/j.iccl.2020.05.001
2211-7458/20/© 2020 Elsevier Inc. All rights reserved.

physiology evaluation to guide revascularization.[11,12] In the present report, the authors review the application of FFR spanning from early efforts to the FAME trials to current practice and address controversies related to these trials, barriers to uptake of FFR, and future directions in the domain of FFR and coronary physiology-based revascularization.

HISTORICAL BACKGROUND

Before the advent of percutaneous transluminal coronary angioplasty (PTCA), laboratory studies demonstrated that coronary flow reserve (CFR), defined as the ratio of maximal coronary flow during hyperemia to resting coronary flow, was inversely related to progressive epicardial stenosis.[13] Indeed, Grüntzig and colleagues[14] applied these mechanistic insights to gauge the efficacy of the first human PTCA in 1977 by measuring the residual resting pressure gradient (proportional to flow) across the treated stenosis. However, these efforts were limited by several factors, including the lack of hyperemic assessment and the overestimation of gradients owing to the size of end-hole catheters used to calculate distal pressure. Consequently, the early era of PCI was defined by an angiography-only strategy for revascularization using noninvasive stress imaging modalities and/or visual estimation of angiographic stenoses to localize ischemia, followed by measurement of Doppler wire–derived CFR. However, frustration with the handling characteristics of the Doppler wire, realization of the limitations of CFR, the development of a coronary pressure wire in the early 1990s, and the description and validation of FFR by Pijls and De Bruyne launched the revolution bringing the invasive assessment of coronary physiology to the forefront of PCI.

FRACTIONAL FLOW RESERVE
Definition
FFR is defined as the ratio of maximal myocardial blood flow in the presence of an epicardial coronary stenosis to normal maximal flow (ie, in the theoretic absence of the stenosis). Derived from Ohm's law, myocardial flow equals the change in pressure across the microvasculature (ie, distal coronary pressure minus central venous pressure) divided by the resistance of entire coronary tree. A few fundamental assumptions simplify this calculation and establish that myocardial flow is proportional to coronary pressure, namely that (1) venous pressure is negligible compared with coronary pressure, and (2) epicardial and

microvascular coronary resistance is minimized by the vasodilators nitroglycerin and adenosine, respectively. In a stenotic vessel, the aortic pressure reflects what the distal coronary pressure would be in the absence of disease. Taken together, FFR equals the mean distal coronary pressure divided by the mean aortic pressure at maximal hyperemia and thus represents the proportion of normal flow reaching the myocardial territory subtended by the interrogated vessel. Importantly, therefore, the derivation of FFR illustrates many of its distinct attributes, namely, that FFR is specific to the epicardial vessel, is highly reproducible, and has a normal value of 1.0 in every vessel per patient.[15]

Validation
In 1996, Pijls and colleagues[10] published the seminal trial validating FFR in 45 patients with stable angina and angiographically intermediate stenoses. Because there was no consensus gold-standard noninvasive stress test for the diagnosis of ischemia, the investigators combined bicycle exercise testing, stress echocardiography, and thallium scintigraphy to create a reference standard with greater than 95% diagnostic accuracy. Compared with this reference standard, an FFR threshold of less than 0.75 conferred a diagnostic accuracy of 93% for ischemia (sensitivity 88%, specificity 100%). Subsequently, the seminal Deferral versus Performance of PCI of Non-Ischemia Producing Stenoses (DEFER) trial published in 2001 demonstrated the safety of deferring revascularization of stenoses with FFR values ≥0.75 and recently reported 15-year data were consistent without evidence of a late catch-up phenomenon (Fig. 1).[5,16] Additional studies demonstrated that extending the ischemic threshold from less than 0.75 to ≤0.80 improved sensitivity without meaningfully affecting specificity.[17] It is with this backdrop of safely deferring revascularization for nonischemic FFR values that the FAME investigators embarked on the landmark FAME trials.

FRACTIONAL FLOW RESERVE VERSUS ANGIOGRAPHY FOR MULTIVESSEL EVALUATION TRIAL: FRACTIONAL FLOW RESERVE VERSUS ANGIOGRAPHY FOR GUIDING PERCUTANEOUS CORONARY INTERVENTION
Study Design
Published in 2009, FAME was a multicenter, international, randomized clinical trial in 1005 patients with multivessel coronary artery disease (CAD) (≥50% diameter stenosis in at least 2

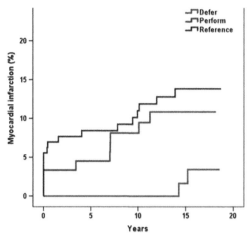

Fig. 1. Kaplan-Meier analysis of MI at 15-year follow-up stratified by treatment strategy. The deferral of revascularization of stenoses with FFR values ≥0.75 was associated with long-term safety without a late catch-up phenomenon. Defer: no PCI for FFR ≥0.75; perform: PCI for FFR ≥0.75; reference: PCI for FFR less than 0.75. (*Adapted from* Zimmermann FM, Ferrara A, Johnson NP, et al. Deferral vs. performance of percutaneous coronary intervention of functionally non-significant coronary stenosis: 15-year follow-up of the DEFER trial. Eur. Heart J. 2015;36:3182–3188; with permission.)

major epicardial vessels) undergoing PCI that compared an FFR-guided strategy with the standard angiography-guided strategy.[11] Key exclusion criteria included significant left main disease or disease in which coronary artery bypass surgery (CABG) was determined to be the preferred treatment, prior CABG, extremely tortuous or calcified vessels, recent (<5 days) ST-segment elevation myocardial infarction (STEMI), and cardiogenic shock. In the FFR group, PCI was only performed for stenoses with FFR values ≤0.80. The primary endpoint was the composite of death, myocardial infarction (MI), or repeat revascularization at 1 year.

Primary Results
Baseline clinical characteristics among the angiography-only (N = 496) and FFR (N = 509) groups were similar. Two-thirds of the overall cohort had stable ischemic heart disease (SIHD), whereas the remaining one-third presented with unstable angina or non-ST-segment elevation myocardial infarction (NSTEMI). On angiography, there were no significant between-group differences in the mean number of significant stenoses per patient (2.7 ± 0.9 vs 2.8 ± 1.0) or intermediate (50%–70% diameter stenosis), severe (71%–90% diameter stenosis), or critical (91%–100% diameter stenosis) stenoses (41% vs 44%, 41% vs 38%, and

18% vs 18%, respectively). In the FFR group, 63% of the angiographically significant stenoses had an FFR ≤0.80 (35% of intermediate, 80% of severe, and 96% of critical stenoses). Consequently, there were significantly more stents per patient placed in the angiography-only group (2.7 ± 1.2 vs 1.9 ± 1.3, $P<.001$). The procedure time was similar between groups, but the angiography-only group received significantly more contrast volume (302 ± 127 mL vs 272 ± 133 mL, $P<.001$).

The primary endpoint occurred significantly more often in the angiography-only group compared with the FFR group at 1 year (18.3% vs 13.2%, $P = .02$). This finding was driven by numerically lower event rates across each of the individual component endpoints (death, MI, and repeat revascularization) (Fig. 2). Furthermore, the secondary endpoint of death or MI also occurred at a significantly increased rate in the angiography-only group (11.1% vs 7.3%, $P = .04$). Angina-free survival at 1 year was similar between groups (78% vs 81%).

Longer-Term Data
At 2 years, the primary endpoint continued to occur more frequently in the angiography-only group compared with the FFR group, although the difference did not reach statistical significance (22% vs 18%, $P = .08$). However, the rate of death or MI remained significantly higher in the angiography-only group (13% vs 8%, $P = .02$).[18] At 5 years, these differences in the rates of the primary endpoint (31% vs 28%, $P = .31$) and death or MI (20% vs 17%, $P = .24$) were more modest.[19]

Cost-Effectiveness
The mean cost of the index procedure was significantly higher in the angiography group than the FFR group ($6007 ± $2819 vs $5332 ± $3261, $P<.001$). A dedicated cost-effectiveness analysis suggested that FFR-guided PCI in multivessel CAD was a dominant strategy; that is, it was one that not only improved clinical outcomes but also provided cost savings (Fig. 3).[20]

FRACTIONAL FLOW RESERVE VERSUS ANGIOGRAPHY FOR MULTIVESSEL EVALUATION 2 TRIAL: FRACTIONAL FLOW RESERVE-GUIDED PERCUTANEOUS CORONARY INTERVENTION VERSUS MEDICAL THERAPY IN STABLE CORONARY DISEASE
Study Design
One of the criticisms of the original FAME trial was that there was not an arm that received

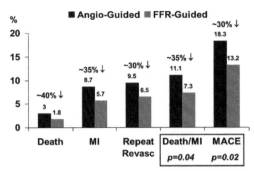

Fig. 2. Outcomes at 1 year among patients randomized to FFR-guided versus angiography-guided PCI in FAME. FFR-guided PCI was associated with a 30% to 40% relative risk reduction in individual major adverse cardiac event endpoints, including significantly less death or MI.

optimal medical therapy (OMT) alone. FAME 2 sought to answer the question of whether PCI improved outcomes when compared with OMT in patients with SIHD. FAME 2 was a multicenter, international, randomized clinical trial published in 2012 that compared the initial strategies of FFR-guided PCI with OMT in 1220 patients with SIHD.[12] All patients underwent coronary angiography and FFR interrogation of all ≥50% diameter stenoses deemed by the operator to require stenting based on angiographic and clinical data. Patients with at least 1 functionally

significant stenosis (FFR ≤0.80) were randomized to FFR-guided PCI versus OMT, whereas those whose stenoses all had FFR values greater than 0.80 were enrolled in a registry and also treated with OMT. OMT consisted of at least an aspirin, beta-blocker, angiotensin-converting enzyme inhibitor or angiotensin II receptor blocker, and statin therapy. Important exclusion criteria included recent (<1 week) acute coronary syndrome (ACS), significant left main disease or multivessel CAD in which CABG was considered the preferred treatment, prior CABG, and extremely tortuous or calcified vessels. The primary endpoint was the composite of death, MI, or urgent revascularization at 2 years.

Primary Results

Baseline clinical characteristics among the FFR-guided PCI (N = 447), OMT (N = 441), and registry (N = 166) groups were largely similar, and nearly 70% of the overall cohort had class II–IV Canadian Cardiovascular Society scale angina. In comparison to the registry cohort, the randomized groups had significantly more total stenoses per patient and angiographically severe stenoses per patient. The number of functionally significant stenoses per patient was similar in the FFR-guided PCI and OMT groups (1.52 ± 0.78 vs 1.42 ± 0.73), including the subset of those

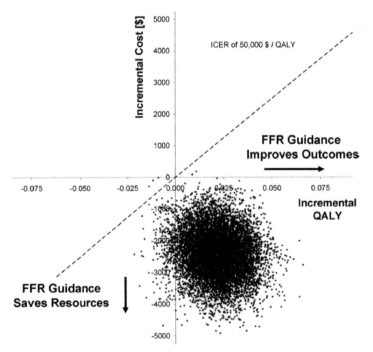

Fig. 3. Cost-effectiveness model of FFR-guided versus angiography-guided PCI in FAME. Compared with angiography-guided PCI, FFR-guided PCI was associated with more incremental QALYs (denotes greater efficacy) and negative incremental costs (denotes greater cost savings). QALY; quality-adjusted life-year. (From Fearon WF, Bornschein B, Tonino PAL, et al. Economic evaluation of fractional flow reserve-guided percutaneous coronary intervention in patients with multivessel disease. Circulation 2010;122:2545–2550; with permission.)

located in the proximal or midsegment of the left anterior descending coronary artery (62% vs 60%).

Patient recruitment was stopped prematurely by the independent Data and Safety Monitoring Board because of a significantly lower rate of the primary endpoint in the FFR-guided PCI group compared with the OMT group (4.3% vs 12.7%, hazard ratio [HR] = 0.32, 95% confidence interval [CI]: 0.19–0.53; P<.001). This difference at short-term follow-up (213 ± 128 days) was driven by substantially less urgent revascularization (1.6% vs 11.1%; HR = 0.13; 95% CI: 0.06–0.30; P<.001) in the FFR-guided PCI group, particularly those prompted by MI or ischemic electrocardiographic changes. There were no significant between-group differences in the rates of death or MI. Among patients in the registry cohort, the rate of the primary endpoint was 3%.

Longer-Term Data

The rate of the primary endpoint remained significantly lower in the FFR-guided PCI group compared with the OMT group at 2 years (8.1% vs 19.5%, HR = 0.39, 95% CI: 0.26–0.57; P<.001), 3 years, and 5 years (13.9% vs 27%, HR = 0.46, 95% CI: 0.34–0.63; P<.001), owing to a sustained reduction in urgent revascularizations over time.[21] At 5 years, there remained no significant between-group differences in MI or death. However, overall MI and spontaneous MI were both lower in the FFR-guided PCI arm compared with OMT alone (Fig. 4). The FFR-guided group did experience a significantly greater relief from angina at 3 years, although this difference was less pronounced at 5 years, by which time 51% of OMT group had crossed over and underwent revascularization. The rate of the primary endpoint was similar between the FFR-guided PCI group and the registry cohort at 5-year follow-up (13.9% vs 15.7%).[22]

Cost-Effectiveness

As expected, the mean baseline cost was substantially higher in the FFR-guided PCI group than the OMT group because of PCI-related costs ($9944 vs $4440, P<.001). However, because of the increased number of urgent revascularizations and other adverse cardiac events, costs were similar between the groups by 3-year follow-up ($16,792 vs $16,737, P = .94). Cost-effectiveness analyses at 3 years showed that FFR-guided PCI provided a favorable incremental cost-effectiveness ratio of $1600 per quality-adjusted life-year.[23]

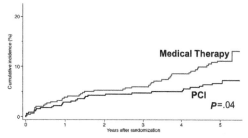

PCI vs. Medical Therapy: HR 0.62 (95% CI 0.39-0.99)

Fig. 4. Kaplan-Meier analysis of spontaneous MI at 5-year follow-up stratified by FFR-guided PCI versus OMT in FAME 2. There were significantly less spontaneous MIs among those who underwent FFR-guided PCI compared with those who received OMT. (*Adapted from* Xaplanteris P, Fournier S, Pijls NHJ, et al. Five-Year Outcomes with PCI Guided by Fractional Flow Reserve. N. Engl. J. Med. 2018;379:250–259; with permission.)

DISCUSSION

The salient findings from the landmark FAME trials in patients with predominantly SIHD were that an initial FFR-guided strategy for PCI significantly improved clinical outcomes compared with the initial strategies of angiography-only PCI or OMT alone. These pivotal data established the clinical efficacy, safety, and cost-effectiveness of an FFR-directed strategy for PCI. Taken together with the findings from DEFER, the FAME trials paved the way for the current era of coronary physiology-guided revascularization over the past decade. Indeed, the latest American College of Cardiology/American Heart Association and European Society of Cardiology guidelines and appropriate use criteria (AUC) reflect these randomized data and recommend the use of FFR in SIHD to achieve functionally complete revascularization.[24–27]

Controversies

Despite a strong endorsement from major societal guidelines and AUC, there remain some controversial aspects of the FAME trials that are worth considering. First, critics argue that the FFR threshold for functionally significant ischemia in the FAME trials should have been less than 0.75 as established in the DEFER trial rather than ≤0.80. As described earlier, previous studies have shown that raising the threshold from less than 0.75 to ≤0.80 led to higher sensitivity without appreciably lowering specificity, and so the FAME investigators chose the upper limit of this ischemic transition zone in order to treat the most number of ischemia-producing stenoses.[17] Data from subsequent studies have supported the notion of an ischemic gray zone, that is, although FFR values less than 0.75 indicate functionally significant ischemia that should be treated, and values greater than 0.80 indicate nonsignificant ischemia that can safely be managed with OMT, intermediate values from 0.75 to 0.80 represent a gray zone in which additional clinical features should be considered to determine if revascularization is warranted.[28] Second, the early termination of enrollment in FAME 2 has been criticized because it (1) may have exaggerated treatment effects, and (2) reduced the ability to detect differences in the rates of hard outcomes (ie, death and MI) between the FFR-guided PCI and OMT groups.[29] Nonetheless, given the large between-group difference in the primary outcome in short-term follow-up and the strong recommendation of the independent Data and Safety Monitoring Board to halt enrollment, the investigators concluded that further patient recruitment would have been inappropriate.

Finally, despite blinded adjudication of events, the possibility that physician/patient awareness of a functionally significant stenosis influenced the rate of urgent revascularizations in the OMT group of FAME 2 has been touted as a major limitation. However, patients in the registry cohort with angiographically significant stenoses had a substantially lower rate of the primary outcome compared with the OMT group, suggesting that physician/patient awareness of an untreated stenosis alone cannot explain the increased number of urgent revascularizations in the OMT group. In addition, the fact that the number urgent revascularizations triggered by objective data (ie, MI or ischemic electrocardiographic changes) was higher in the OMT group than the FFR-guided PCI group further mitigates this perceived controversy. A subsequent study looked at the effect of PCI on quality of life in SIHD patients enrolled in the FAME trials and found that it improved to a greater degree in patients with lower FFR values and/or a larger change in FFR from pre-PCI to post-PCI,[30] which suggests that the degree of ischemia dictated the improvement in symptoms and that it was not due to knowledge of having undergone PCI. If the improvement had only been due to a placebo effect, then all patients would have improved to a similar degree. Finally, an analysis of outcomes in the OMT arm of FAME 2 showed a very clear relationship between the FFR value and the rate of outcomes, again arguing that it was not the knowledge of not receiving a stent that drove outcomes (Fig. 5).[31]

Temporal Trends

Following the publication of FAME and FAME 2, several registry-based studies reported consistent findings of improved clinical outcomes with an FFR-based approach to PCI.[32–34] However, despite these robust randomized and real-world data as well as recommendation from major societal guidelines, FFR remains underused. Early data from the National Cardiovascular Data Registry CathPCI Registry revealed that the rate of FFR use among nearly 400,000 patients with angiographically intermediate SIHD who underwent PCI increased from 8% in 2009 to only 34% in 2014.[35] In a similar patient population, a more recent Veterans Affairs (VA) registry-based study reported an FFR-guided PCI rate of 62% in 2014 that increased to 75% in 2017. Although this discordance may reflect fundamental differences between the VA and NCDR sites (ie, the VA Healthcare System has a greater degree of academic affiliation and lacks fee-for-service reimbursement), it also points to the phenomenon of real-world lag in practice following release of trial data and clinical guidelines. Notably, among all-comers with angiographically intermediate SIHD, which also captures patients who had PCI deferred based on FFR values in the nonischemic range, the rates of FFR use over time in this VA-based cohort were much more modest, incrementally increasing from 15% in 2009 to 19% in 2017.[36]

Barriers to Adoption

Several factors have been cited as impediments to the more widespread use of FFR, including time, poor reimbursement, and the need for hyperemia. The perception that measuring FFR

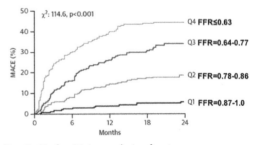

Fig. 5. Kaplan-Meier analysis of outcomes among patients treated with OMT in FAME 2 stratified by FFR values. The lower the FFR values, the greater the degree of ischemia and the higher the event rates. (*Adapted from* Barbato E, Toth GG, Johnson NP, et al. A Prospective Natural History Study of Coronary Atherosclerosis Using Fractional Flow Reserve. J. Am. Coll. Cardiol. 2016;68:2247–2255; with permission.)

lengthens procedural times is founded in operator belief regarding the need for PCI (ie, cases with stenoses that do not warrant PCI are prolonged by FFR interrogation). However, as shown in FAME, these cases are offset by those in which the operator deems PCI to be necessary, but the FFR value falls in the nonischemic range and stenting is averted, shortening procedural times. Prior studies have also implicated poor operator financial incentives as a cause of FFR underutilization, and this notion was substantiated by a published survey of operators.[37,38] The perceived detriment of adenosine-induced hyperemia has led to the emergence of nonhyperemic pressure ratios, and in doing so, has effectively eliminated hyperemia as a barrier to the invasive assessment of coronary physiology.[39,40]

The lack of survival benefit with an FFR-guided strategy in the FAME trials has also been referenced as a reason to dismiss FFR. This mindset devalues other important endpoints for patients, including relief from angina and avoidance of urgent revascularization, let alone key health care quality-related metrics, such as inappropriate PCI and cost-effectiveness. However, the recent VA registry-based study in unselected patients with angiographically intermediate SIHD reported a 43% lower adjusted risk of death at 1 year with an FFR-guided versus angiography-only revascularization approach, providing hard outcome data in support of FFR, albeit with the limitations of unmeasured confounding inherent to observational data. More interestingly, despite the strong academic ties and fixed payment model that define the VA Healthcare System, and even after adjusting for patient, procedural, and site-level factors, significant site-level variation in FFR utilization was still detected.[36] Coupled with the finding that a negative stress test did not impact FFR use, these sobering data suggest that FFR underuse in current practice arises from operator belief regarding the utility of invasive coronary physiology and that changes to educational training or reimbursement policies would unlikely influence the adoption of FFR.

Future Directions

Notwithstanding the previously described barriers to FFR utilization, the authors expect the use of FFR, and coronary physiology-guided revascularization overall, to steadily increase in the coming decade. First, a series of recent randomized clinical trials have reported improved

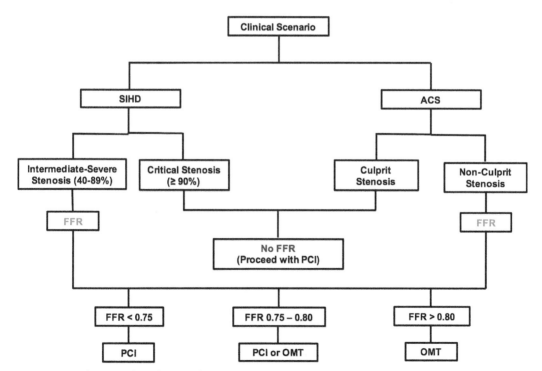

Fig. 6. Approach to FFR-based revascularization in contemporary practice. Algorithm for implementation and interpretation of FFR-guided assessment of coronary stenoses across the spectrum of CAD.

outcomes with an FFR-based approach to revascularization of nonculprit stenoses in the setting of both STEMI and NSTEMI.[41–43] The use of FFR in ACS is already supported by the current AUC and is anticipated to be endorsed by the next updated iteration of ACS guidelines.[27] Second, the application of FFR may further expand based on the forthcoming results of FAME 3, a multicenter, international, randomized clinical trial comparing FFR-guided PCI with CABG in multivessel CAD; patient enrollment into the trial is complete, and the initial data are expected to be published in 2021.[44] Third, the continued alignment of PCI reimbursement policies with AUC and cost-effectiveness will probably lead to increased use of FFR, particularly in SIHD. Last, the authors anticipate that the recent development and validation of alternative indices of coronary physiology, including nonhyperemic pressure ratios (eg, instantaneous wave-free and resting full-cycle ratios), computed tomography–derived FFR, and angiogram-derived FFR, will likely result in greater uptake of coronary physiology–based revascularization.[39,40,45,46]

SUMMARY

FFR overcomes the primary limitation of invasive coronary angiography by accurately localizing which epicardial stenoses cause ischemia and warrant revascularization. The pivotal FAME trials of the last decade established the clinical utility of measuring FFR to direct PCI in patients with predominantly SIHD and ushered in the contemporary era of coronary physiology-guided revascularization. The application of an FFR-guided revascularization strategy is backed by current SIHD guidelines and is expected to expand to nonculprit stenoses in the next update of ACS guidelines based on recent encouraging randomized controlled trial data. Taken together, the authors propose the algorithm for FFR-directed revascularization in current practice shown in **Fig. 6**. The adoption of FFR and other coronary physiologic modalities to guide revascularization will continue to grow over time and define the modern era of revascularization.

DISCLOSURE

W.F. Fearon receives research support from Abbott Vascular and Medtronic, and has minor stock options with HeartFlow and consults for CathWorks. R.V. Parikh has no relationships with industry relevant to the contents of this article to disclose.

REFERENCES

1. Beller GA, Zaret BL. Contributions of nuclear cardiology to diagnosis and prognosis of patients with coronary artery disease. Circulation 2000;101: 1465–78.
2. Hachamovitch R, Berman DS, Shaw LJ, et al. Incremental prognostic value of myocardial perfusion single photon emission computed tomography for the prediction of cardiac death: differential stratification for risk of cardiac death and myocardial infarction. Circulation 1998;97: 535–43.
3. Davies RF, Goldberg AD, Forman S, et al. Asymptomatic Cardiac Ischemia Pilot (ACIP) study two-year follow-up: outcomes of patients randomized to initial strategies of medical therapy versus revascularization. Circulation 1997;95:2037–43.
4. Shaw LJ, Berman DS, Maron DJ, et al. Optimal medical therapy with or without percutaneous coronary intervention to reduce ischemic burden: results from the Clinical Outcomes Utilizing Revascularization and Aggressive Drug Evaluation (COURAGE) trial nuclear substudy. Circulation 2008;117:1283–91.
5. Bech GJ, De Bruyne B, Pijls NH, et al. Fractional flow reserve to determine the appropriateness of angioplasty in moderate coronary stenosis: a randomized trial. Circulation 2001;103:2928–34.
6. Boden WE, O'Rourke RA, Teo KK, et al. Optimal medical therapy with or without PCI for stable coronary disease. N Engl J Med 2007;356: 1503–16.
7. Fischer JJ, Samady H, McPherson JA, et al. Comparison between visual assessment and quantitative angiography versus fractional flow reserve for native coronary narrowings of moderate severity. Am J Cardiol 2002;90:210–5.
8. Tonino PAL, Fearon WF, De Bruyne B, et al. Angiographic versus functional severity of coronary artery stenoses in the FAME study fractional flow reserve versus angiography in multivessel evaluation. J Am Coll Cardiol 2010;55:2816–21.
9. Lima RSL, Watson DD, Goode AR, et al. Incremental value of combined perfusion and function over perfusion alone by gated SPECT myocardial perfusion imaging for detection of severe three-vessel coronary artery disease. J Am Coll Cardiol 2003; 42:64–70.
10. Pijls NH, De Bruyne B, Peels K, et al. Measurement of fractional flow reserve to assess the functional severity of coronary-artery stenoses. N Engl J Med 1996;334:1703–8.
11. Tonino PAL, De Bruyne B, Pijls NHJ, et al. Fractional flow reserve versus angiography for guiding percutaneous coronary intervention. N Engl J Med 2009;360:213–24.

12. De Bruyne B, Pijls NHJ, Kalesan B, et al. Fractional flow reserve-guided PCI versus medical therapy in stable coronary disease. N Engl J Med 2012;367: 991–1001.

13. Gould KL, Lipscomb K, Hamilton GW. Physiologic basis for assessing critical coronary stenosis. Instantaneous flow response and regional distribution during coronary hyperemia as measures of coronary flow reserve. Am J Cardiol 1974;33: 87–94.

14. Grüntzig AR, Senning A, Siegenthaler WE. Nonoperative dilatation of coronary-artery stenosis: percutaneous transluminal coronary angioplasty. N Engl J Med 1979;301:61–8.

15. Pijls NH, van Son JA, Kirkeeide RL, et al. Experimental basis of determining maximum coronary, myocardial, and collateral blood flow by pressure measurements for assessing functional stenosis severity before and after percutaneous transluminal coronary angioplasty. Circulation 1993;87: 1354–67.

16. Zimmermann FM, Ferrara A, Johnson NP, et al. Deferral vs. performance of percutaneous coronary intervention of functionally non-significant coronary stenosis: 15-year follow-up of the DEFER trial. Eur Heart J 2015;36:3182–8.

17. De Bruyne B, Pijls NH, Bartunek J, et al. Fractional flow reserve in patients with prior myocardial infarction. Circulation 2001;104:157–62.

18. Pijls NHJ, Fearon WF, Tonino PAL, et al. Fractional flow reserve versus angiography for guiding percutaneous coronary intervention in patients with multivessel coronary artery disease: 2-year follow-up of the FAME (Fractional Flow Reserve Versus Angiography for Multivessel Evaluation) study. J Am Coll Cardiol 2010;56:177–84.

19. van Nunen LX, Zimmermann FM, Tonino PAL, et al. Fractional flow reserve versus angiography for guidance of PCI in patients with multivessel coronary artery disease (FAME): 5-year follow-up of a randomised controlled trial. Lancet 2015;386: 1853–60.

20. Fearon WF, Bornschein B, Tonino PAL, et al. Economic evaluation of fractional flow reserve-guided percutaneous coronary intervention in patients with multivessel disease. Circulation 2010;122: 2545–50.

21. De Bruyne B, Fearon WF, Pijls NHJ, et al. Fractional flow reserve-guided PCI for stable coronary artery disease. N Engl J Med 2014;371:1208–17.

22. Xaplanteris P, Fournier S, Pijls NHJ, et al. Five-year outcomes with PCI guided by fractional flow reserve. N Engl J Med 2018;379:250–9.

23. Fearon WF, Nishi T, De Bruyne B, et al. Clinical outcomes and cost-effectiveness of fractional flow reserve-guided percutaneous coronary intervention in patients with stable coronary artery disease: three-year follow-up of the FAME 2 trial (fractional flow reserve versus angiography for multivessel evaluation). Circulation 2018;137:480–7.

24. Fihn SD, Blankenship JC, Alexander KP, et al. 2014 ACC/AHA/AATS/PCNA/SCAI/STS focused update of the guideline for the diagnosis and management of patients with stable ischemic heart disease. Circulation 2014;130:1749–67.

25. Knuuti J, Wijns W, Saraste A, et al. 2019 ESC Guidelines for the diagnosis and management of chronic coronary syndromes. Eur Heart J 2020;41: 407–77.

26. Patel MR, Calhoon JH, Dehmer GJ, et al. ACC/AATS/AHA/ASE/ASNC/SCAI/SCCT/STS 2017 appropriate use criteria for coronary revascularization in patients with stable ischemic heart disease: a report of the American College of Cardiology Appropriate Use Criteria Task Force, American Association for Thoracic Surgery, American Heart Association, American Society of Echocardiography, American Society of Nuclear Cardiology, Society for Cardiovascular Angiography and Interventions, Society of Cardiovascular Computed Tomography, and Society of Thoracic Surgeons. J Am Coll Cardiol 2017;69:2212–41.

27. Patel MR, Calhoon JH, Dehmer GJ, et al. ACC/AATS/AHA/ASE/ASNC/SCAI/SCCT/STS 2016 appropriate use criteria for coronary revascularization in patients with acute coronary syndromes: a report of the American College of Cardiology Appropriate Use Criteria Task Force, American Association for Thoracic Surgery, American Heart Association, American Society of Echocardiography, American Society of Nuclear Cardiology, Society for Cardiovascular Angiography and Interventions, Society of Cardiovascular Computed Tomography, and the Society of Thoracic Surgeons. J Am Coll Cardiol 2017;69:570–91.

28. Adjedj J, De Bruyne B, Floré V, et al. Significance of intermediate values of fractional flow reserve in patients with coronary artery disease. Circulation 2016;133:502–8.

29. Bassler D, Briel M, Montori VM, et al. Stopping randomized trials early for benefit and estimation of treatment effects: systematic review and meta-regression analysis. JAMA 2010;303:1180–7.

30. Nishi T, Piroth Z, De Bruyne B, et al. Fractional flow reserve and quality-of-life improvement after percutaneous coronary intervention in patients with stable coronary artery disease. Circulation 2018;138:1797–804.

31. Barbato E, Toth GG, Johnson NP, et al. A prospective natural history study of coronary atherosclerosis using fractional flow reserve. J Am Coll Cardiol 2016;68:2247–55.

32. Park S-J, Ahn J-M, Park G-M, et al. Trends in the outcomes of percutaneous coronary intervention with

the routine incorporation of fractional flow reserve in real practice. Eur Heart J 2013;34:3353–61.

33. Li J, Elrashidi MY, Flammer AJ, et al. Long-term outcomes of fractional flow reserve-guided vs. angiography-guided percutaneous coronary intervention in contemporary practice. Eur Heart J 2013;34:1375–83.

34. Van Belle E, Rioufol G, Pouillot C, et al. Outcome impact of coronary revascularization strategy reclassification with fractional flow reserve at time of diagnostic angiography: insights from a large French multicenter fractional flow reserve registry. Circulation 2014;129:173–85.

35. Desai NR, Bradley SM, Parzynski CS, et al. Appropriate use criteria for coronary revascularization and trends in utilization, patient selection, and appropriateness of percutaneous coronary intervention. JAMA 2015;314:2045–53.

36. Parikh RV, Liu G, Plomondon ME, et al. Utilization and outcomes of measuring fractional flow reserve in patients with stable ischemic heart disease. J Am Coll Cardiol 2020;75:409–19.

37. Dattilo PB, Prasad A, Honeycutt E, et al. Contemporary patterns of fractional flow reserve and intravascular ultrasound use among patients undergoing percutaneous coronary intervention in the United States: insights from the National Cardiovascular Data Registry. J Am Coll Cardiol 2012; 60:2337–9.

38. Hannawi B, Lam WW, Wang S, et al. Current use of fractional flow reserve: a nationwide survey. Tex Heart Inst J 2014;41:579–84.

39. Sen S, Escaned J, Malik IS, et al. Development and validation of a new adenosine-independent index of stenosis severity from coronary wave-intensity analysis: results of the ADVISE (ADenosine Vasodilator Independent Stenosis Evaluation) study. J Am Coll Cardiol 2012;59:1392–402.

40. Svanerud J, Ahn J-M, Jeremias A, et al. Validation of a novel non-hyperaemic index of coronary artery stenosis severity: the Resting Full-cycle Ratio (VALIDATE RFR) study. EuroIntervention 2018;14:806–14.

41. Engstrøm T, Kelbæk H, Helqvist S, et al. Complete revascularisation versus treatment of the culprit lesion only in patients with ST-segment elevation myocardial infarction and multivessel disease (DANAMI-3—PRIMULTI): an open-label, randomised controlled trial. Lancet 2015;386: 665–71.

42. Layland J, Oldroyd KG, Curzen N, et al. Fractional flow reserve vs. angiography in guiding management to optimize outcomes in non-ST-segment elevation myocardial infarction: the British Heart Foundation FAMOUS-NSTEMI randomized trial. Eur Heart J 2015;36:100–11.

43. Smit M, Brinkman K, Geerlings S, et al. Future challenges for clinical care of an ageing population infected with HIV: a modelling study. Lancet Infect Dis 2015;15:810–8.

44. Zimmermann FM, De Bruyne B, Pijls NHJ, et al. Rationale and design of the Fractional Flow Reserve versus Angiography for Multivessel Evaluation (FAME) 3 Trial: a comparison of fractional flow reserve-guided percutaneous coronary intervention and coronary artery bypass graft surgery in patients with multivessel coronary artery disease. Am Heart J 2015;170:619–26.e2.

45. Koo B-K, Erglis A, Doh J-H, et al. Diagnosis of ischemia-causing coronary stenoses by noninvasive fractional flow reserve computed from coronary computed tomographic angiograms. Results from the prospective multicenter DISCOVER-FLOW (Diagnosis of Ischemia-Causing Stenoses Obtained Via Noninvasive Fractional Flow Reserve) study. J Am Coll Cardiol 2011;58:1989–97.

46. Witberg G, De Bruyne B, Fearon WF, et al. Diagnostic performance of angiogram-derived fractional flow reserve: a pooled analysis of 5 prospective cohort studies. JACC Cardiovasc Interv 2020;13(4):488–97.

Percutaneous Coronary Intervention or Surgery for Unprotected Left Main Disease
EXCEL Trial at 5 Years

Lorenzo Azzalini, MD, PhD, MSc[a],
Gregg W. Stone, MD[a,b,*]

KEYWORDS

- Left main • Coronary artery disease • Percutaneous coronary intervention
- Coronary artery bypass graft • PCI • CABG • Revascularization • EXCEL

KEY POINTS

- The Evaluation of XIENCE versus Coronary Artery Bypass Surgery for Effectiveness of Left Main Revascularization (EXCEL) trial compared the outcomes of patients with left main coronary artery disease of low or intermediate anatomic complexity undergoing revascularization with percutaneous coronary intervention (PCI) with everolimus-eluting stents versus coronary artery bypass graft (CABG).
- The primary endpoint of all-cause death, stroke, or myocardial infarction at a median 3-year follow-up occurred with similar frequency in the 2 study arms, and PCI met study criteria for noninferiority compared with CABG.
- Extended follow-up at 5 years showed that there still was no significant difference between PCI and CABG with regard to the rates of the primary endpoint.
- During the first 30 days after revascularization, PCI was associated with a lower risk of the primary endpoint. Between 30 days and 1 year, there were similar adverse event rates between PCI and CABG. Between 1 year and 5 years, the risk for the primary endpoint was higher in the PCI arm. The mean event-free survival time through 5 years was similar after PCI and CABG.
- At present, PCI may be considered an appropriate alternative to CABG in selected patients with left main disease and low or intermediate anatomic complexity (site-assessed Synergy Between PCI with Taxus and Cardiac Surgery [SYNTAX] score ≤32).

BACKGROUND

Left main (LM) coronary artery disease (CAD) is present in up to 6% of patients who undergo coronary angiography[1] and in 12% of subjects presenting with acute coronary syndromes.[2] It is associated with multivessel CAD in approximately 70% of cases.[3,4] LM disease is associated with a poor prognosis with medical therapy, given the large myocardial territory at risk (ranging from 75% to 100% of the myocardium depending on the coronary dominance). Revascularization is recommended by current guidelines for patients with an LM stenosis greater than or equal to

---

Funding: The EXCEL trial was funded by Abbott Vascular, Santa Clara, CA. There was no funding for this article.
[a] The Zena and Michael A. Wiener Cardiovascular Institute, Icahn School of Medicine at Mount Sinai, 1 Gustave L. Levy Place, New York, NY 10029, USA; [b] The Cardiovascular Research Foundation, New York, NY, USA
* Corresponding author. Mount Sinai Hospital, Cardiovascular Research Foundation, 1700 Broadway, 8th Floor, New York, NY 10019.
E-mail address: gregg.stone@mountsinai.org
Twitter: @lorenzo2509 (L.A.); @GreggWStone (G.W.S.)

Intervent Cardiol Clin 9 (2020) 419–432
https://doi.org/10.1016/j.iccl.2020.05.002
2211-7458/20/© 2020 Elsevier Inc. All rights reserved.

50%, regardless of symptomatic status or associated ischemic burden.[5,6] This recommendation is based on the high rates of mortality in medically managed patients with severe LM disease (ranging from 20%–30% in low-risk groups to >50% in high-risk patients at 3–4 years)[7,8] and the superiority of LM revascularization compared with medical therapy alone observed in multiple randomized controlled trials (RCTs).[9]

SURGICAL VERSUS PERCUTANEOUS LEFT MAIN REVASCULARIZATION: DATA FROM THE 1990S

Traditionally, coronary artery bypass graft (CABG) surgery has represented the gold standard for LM revascularization.[8–11] The constant advancements in the field of percutaneous coronary intervention (PCI), however, have made feasible a minimally invasive approach to certain groups of patients with LM disease. An individual patient data pooled analysis, including 7812 patients with multivessel disease from 10 RCTs conducted in the 1990s. found no difference in all-cause mortality between CABG and PCI at 5 years (hazard ratio [HR] 0.91; 95% CI, 0.82–1.02; $P = .12$) in the whole population, whereas a benefit of CABG was observed in high-risk groups (such as diabetics and older patients).[12] This report does not reflect, however, the outcomes of contemporary surgical and interventional practices, with suboptimal rates of internal mammary artery use (as low as 39%) and bare metal stents (BMSs) used in 4 of 10 studies.

SYNTAX TRIAL

The development of drug-eluting stent (DES) platforms with reduced failure rates compared with BMSs[13] enhanced the potential of PCI as a competitive revascularization modality compared with CABG in complex CAD. In the landmark Synergy Between PCI with Taxus and Cardiac Surgery (SYNTAX) trial,[4] 1800 patients with 3-vessel or LM CAD were randomized to undergo CABG or PCI with first-generation paclitaxel-eluting stents. The rates of the primary endpoint, major adverse cardiac or cerebrovascular events (MACCEs), a composite of all-cause death, stroke, myocardial infarction (MI), or repeat revascularization, at 12 months, were higher in the PCI group (17.8% vs 12.4%, respectively; $P = .002$), driven by repeat revascularization (13.5% vs 5.9%, respectively; $P<.001$). Consequently, PCI did not meet the prespecified goal for noninferiority. The rates of death

and MI, however, were similar between groups, whereas stroke was more likely to occur with CABG (2.2% vs 0.6%, respectively; $P = .003$). In the prespecified and stratified LM subgroup (n = 705), MACCE rates at 5 years were 36.9% versus 31.0% in PCI versus CABG patients (HR 1.23; 95% CI, 0.95–1.59; $P = .12$). Mortality rates were 12.8% versus 14.6% (HR 0.88; 95% CI, 0.58–1.32; $P = .53$). Stroke was significantly increased in the CABG group (PCI 1.5% vs CABG 4.3%; HR 0.33; 95% CI, 0.12–0.92; $P = .03$), although repeat revascularization was greater in the PCI arm (26.7% vs 15.5%, respectively; HR 1.82; 95% CI, 1.28–2.57; $P<.01$). Importantly, MACCE rates were similar between groups in patients with low and intermediate SYNTAX scores (≤32) but increased in PCI patients with high scores (>32). A recently published extended follow-up report (SYNTAX – Extended Survival)[14] showed no differences in the primary endpoint of 10-year all-cause death between PCI and CABG in patients with LM disease (26% vs 28%, respectively; HR 0.90; 95% CI, 0.68–1.20), whereas PCI was associated with higher mortality in subjects with multivessel CAD (28% vs 21%, respectively; HR 1.41; 95% CI, 1.10–1.80; P for interaction = 0.019). The results of the SYNTAX trial led to the adoption of SYNTAX score calculation in clinical guidelines,[5,6] which now mandate the use of this angiographic tool to inform the decision making regarding revascularization modalities for patients with LM and/or multivessel CAD.

PRECOMBAT AND NOBLE TRIALS

The Premier of Randomized Comparison of Bypass Surgery Versus Angioplasty Using Sirolimus-Eluting Stent in Patients with Left Main Coronary Artery Disease (PRECOMBAT) trial randomized 600 patients with LM stenosis to undergo CABG or PCI with first-generation sirolimus-eluting stents. The 1-year rates of MACCEs (the primary endpoint), a composite of all-cause death, stroke, MI, or ischemia-driven target-vessel revascularization (ID-TVR), were similar between PCI and CABG (8.7% vs 6.7%, respectively; absolute risk difference 2.0% points; 95% CI, −1.6 to 5.6; $P = .01$ for noninferiority). There were no differences in the rates of all-cause death, MI, and stroke. At 2 years, there still were no differences between groups with regard to the primary endpoint (12.2% vs 8.1%, respectively; HR 1.50; 95% CI, 0.90–2.52; $P = .12$). ID-TVR was more frequent, however, in the PCI group than in CABG patients (9.0% vs 4.2%, respectively; HR 2.18; 95% CI,

1.10–4.32; $P = .02$). Extended follow-up of this trial (up to 5 years)[15] confirmed these findings, still showing no differences in MACCEs between PCI and CABG (17.5% vs 14.3%, respectively; HR 1.27; 95% CI, 0.84–1.90; $P = .26$) and higher ID-TVR rates with PCI than with CABG (11.4% vs 5.5%, respectively; HR 2.11%; 95% CI, 1.16–3.84; $P = .012$). Stratification by SYNTAX score tertiles did not find major differences across the CAD spectrum of complexity.

The Nordic-Baltic-British Left Main Revascularization Study (NOBLE) trial[16] compared CABG with PCI using second-generation DESs (mainly intermediate-strut-thickness stainless steel biolimus-eluting stents) among 1201 patients with LM disease. Mean SYNTAX score was approximately 22 in both groups. Five-year estimates of MACCEs were 28% for PCI and 18% for CABG (HR 1.51; 95% CI, 1.13–2.00; $P = .0044$), with PCI failing to meet noninferiority. All-cause mortality was similar (11% vs 9%, respectively; HR 1.08; 95% CI, 0.67–1.74; $P = .84$) between groups, whereas PCI was associated with higher risk of nonperiprocedural MI (6% vs 2%, respectively; HR 2.87; 95% CI, 1.40–5.89; $P = 0.0040$) and any revascularization (15% vs 10%, respectively; HR 1.50; 95% CI, 1.04–2.17; $P = .0304$). There was a trend toward higher risk of stroke with PCI (5% vs 2%, respectively; HR 2.20; 95% CI, 0.91–5.36; $P = .08$) due to the increased incidence of strokes between 1 year and 5 years after PCI, a finding not observed previously and possibly due to chance. Procedural MI, which, in many prior studies has occurred in fewer patients after PCI compared with CABG, was not measured in the NOBLE trial.

EVALUATION OF XIENCE VERSUS CORONARY ARTERY BYPASS SURGERY FOR EFFECTIVENESS OF LEFT MAIN REVASCULARIZATION TRIAL: RATIONALE

One of the major limitations of the aforementioned trials was the inclusion of the need for revascularization in the primary composite endpoint to achieve sufficient statistical power. Although death, MI, and stroke are universally considered "hard clinical endpoints" that are associated with significant impact on longevity and quality of life (QOL), revascularization has a lesser impact on patient well-being.[17–19] No trial was adequately powered to evaluate and compare the relative merits of CABG and PCI for a composite endpoint of death, MI, or stroke in patients undergoing LM revascularization.

Additionally, both interventional cardiology and cardiac surgery practices have evolved

significantly over the past decades. In particular, newer-generation thin-strut DESs were introduced, which have a substantially improved safety and efficacy profile compared with the first-generation platforms used in SYNTAX (paclitaxel-eluting stent) and PRECOMBAT (sirolimus-eluting stent). Specifically, the fluoropolymer-coated cobalt-chromium everolimus-eluting stent has been shown to result in lower rates of stent thrombosis, target lesion/vessel revascularization, MI, major adverse cardiac events, and mortality compared with first-generation DESs.[20–22]

At the same time, CABG techniques and postoperative care also have evolved, leading to improved outcomes, with reduced acute morbidity and mortality.[23] Moreover, with the increased use of multiple arterial grafts (in particular, both internal mammary arteries), bypass graft failure rates have declined further, which in turn may lead to better survival and enhanced QOL.[24,25]

To address these limitations, the Evaluation of XIENCE versus Coronary Artery Bypass Surgery for Effectiveness of Left Main Revascularization (EXCEL) was performed.

EVALUATION OF XIENCE VERSUS CORONARY ARTERY BYPASS SURGERY FOR EFFECTIVENESS OF LEFT MAIN REVASCULARIZATION TRIAL: DESIGN

EXCEL was a prospective, open-label, multicenter, international, RCT including 1905 patients.[19] Subjects with significant LM disease, a site-assessed SYNTAX score equal to less than 32, and local Heart Team consensus that the subject was appropriate for revascularization by both PCI and CABG were consented and randomized in a 1:1 fashion to undergo PCI using cobalt-chromium everolimus-eluting stent (Xience, Abbott Vascular, Santa Clara, California) or CABG. Randomization was stratified by diabetes mellitus, SYNTAX score (<23 vs ≥23), and center.

Significant LM disease was defined as an angiographic stenosis $\geq70\%$, or 50% to 69% with additional evidence of ischemia (eg, on noninvasive testing, minimal luminal area ≤6.0 mm^2 on intravascular ultrasound [IVUS], or fractional flow reserve ≤0.80); alternatively, LM-equivalent disease (Medina bifurcation 0-1-1) with significant disease in both the left anterior descending and circumflex ostia also was accepted for inclusion. Major exclusion criteria were prior CABG, prior LM PCI, prior PCI on another non-LM lesion in the previous year, presence of any clinical/angiographic variable leading the interventional cardiologist/cardiac surgeon to believe that equipoise between CABG and PCI was not present, and SYNTAX score greater than or equal to 33 (as assessed by the local investigators). IVUS use was strongly recommended in the PCI arm. LM PCI technique was left at operator's discretion. The protocol recommended, however, a planned 2-stent technique strategy when the side branch was large (≥3 mm), had significant disease and/or lesion length greater than 5 mm, or when there were other special anatomic considerations (eg, severe angulation or heavy calcification). The planned 2-stent technique could include T-stenting, T-and-protrusion stenting, crush stenting, culotte stenting, or rarely V stenting or Y stenting. The use of kissing balloon inflation after any 2-stent technique was strongly recommended. Dual antiplatelet therapy was recommended for at least 1 year. With regard to surgical aspects in the CABG arm, the use of the left internal mammary artery to anterior descending graft was mandated, and arterial grafts were the preferred conduits for other territories. The right internal mammary artery was the preferred second arterial graft and was recommended to graft the next most important and stenotic coronary artery. Graft patency assessment was strongly recommended, either with transit time Doppler flow measurements or with intraoperative angiography. CABG could be performed with or without the assistance of cardiopulmonary bypass, depending on local expertise.

With regard to laboratory tests, creatine kinase myocardial band (CK-MB) levels had to be used to assess baseline entry criteria and postprocedure myonecrosis. Either CK-MB or troponin I or troponin T levels could be used to assess myonecrosis within 48 hours postprocedure. Twelve-lead electrocardiograms (ECGs) were performed preprocedure, within 24 hours postprocedure, at discharge, and at 1-year follow-up.

The primary endpoint was a 3-year composite rate of death, stroke, or MI, powered for sequential noninferiority and superiority testing (definitions for each component are shown in Table 1). All patients also underwent follow-up at 5 years, with an option for additional follow-up to 10 years. Other endpoints included (among others) target lesion revascularization (TLR), TVR, non-TVR, stent thrombosis, bleeding complications, and a composite of death, MI, stroke, or ischemia-driven revascularization.

All principal analyses were performed in the intent-to-treat population. Assuming a primary endpoint event rate of 11.0% in both treatment arms at 3 years,[15] with 2-year minimum time to follow-up, median time to follow-up 3 years, 8% lost to follow-up at 3 years, a noninferiority margin of 4.2%, and patient accrual time of 29 months, randomizing 1900 subjects (approximately 950 per arm) provided an 80% power to demonstrate noninferiority of PCI to CABG with a 1-sided alpha of 0.025. The original investigators' intention was to randomize 2600 patients, which would have provided 90% power. Because enrollment was slower than anticipated, however, sample size was reduced to 1900 patients for an 80% power. Patients were enrolled between September 29, 2010, and March 6, 2014.

EVALUATION OF XIENCE VERSUS CORONARY ARTERY BYPASS SURGERY FOR EFFECTIVENESS OF LEFT MAIN REVASCULARIZATION TRIAL RESULTS AT THE TIME OF THE PRIMARY ENDPOINT AND 5 YEARS

The EXCEL trial primary endpoint findings were published in 2016.[26] The baseline patient population characteristics (n = 1905) were well balanced between the 2 groups. Mean age was 66 years, 29% were diabetics, and mean left ventricular ejection fraction was 57%. The SYNTAX score according to assessment at local sites was low (≤22) in 60.5% of the patients and intermediate (>22–32) in 39.5% of the patients. According to angiographic core laboratory analysis, however, the SYNTAX score was low in 35.8%, intermediate in 40.0%, and high (≥33) in 24.2% of patients; that is, the extent and complexity of CAD were underestimated by the investigators. Distal LM disease was present in 80.5%, and multivessel CAD was present in 51% of the patients. IVUS was used in 77% of PCIs. In the CABG arm, 99% of patients received at least 1 internal mammary artery. At 3-year follow-up, the primary endpoint of death, MI, or stroke occurred with similar frequency in the PCI and CABG groups (15.4% vs 14.7%, respectively; HR 1.00; 95% CI, 0.79–1.26; P = .98), meeting the noninferiority assumption. Treatment effect for the primary endpoint was consistent across prespecified subgroups, including diabetes. At 30 days, the incidence of the primary endpoint was lower in PCI patients (4.9% vs 7.9%, respectively; HR 0.61; 95% CI, 0.42–

Table 1
Definitions of the components of the primary endpoint in EXCEL

Endpoint	Definition
Death	The cause of death was adjudicated as being due to cardiovascular causes, noncardiovascular causes, or undetermined causes: • Cardiovascular death: sudden cardiac death or death due to acute MI, heart failure, cardiogenic shock, stroke, other cardiovascular causes, or bleeding • Noncardiovascular death: any death with known cause not of cardiac or vascular cause • Undetermined cause of death: not attributable to 1 of the above categories of cardiovascular death or to a noncardiovascular cause. All deaths of undetermined cause are included in the cardiovascular category.

MI	Procedural MI: the occurrence within 72 h after either PCI or CABG of 1 of the following:
	• CK-MB >10× URL
	• CK-MB >5× URL, plus 1 of the following:
	  o New pathologic Q-waves in at least 2 contiguous leads or new persistent left bundle branch block
	  o Angiographically documented graft or native coronary artery occlusion or new severe stenosis with thrombosis and/or diminished epicardial flow
	  o Imaging evidence of new loss of viable myocardium or new regional wall motion abnormality
	Spontaneous MI: the occurrence >72 h after any PCI or CABG of
	• The rise and/or fall of cardiac biomarkers (CK-MB or troponin) >1× URL plus 1 of the following:
	  o ECG changes indicative of new ischemia (ST-segment elevation or depression)
	  o Development of pathologic Q-waves ($\geq$0.04 s in duration and $\geq$1 mm in depth) in $\geq$2 contiguous precordial leads or $\geq$2 adjacent limb leads) on the ECG
	  o Angiographically documented graft or native coronary artery occlusion or new severe stenosis with thrombosis and/or diminished epicardial flow
	  o Imaging evidence of new loss of viable myocardium or new regional wall motion abnormality

Stroke	The rapid onset of a new persistent neurologic deficit attributed to an obstruction in cerebral blood flow and/or cerebral hemorrhage with no apparent nonvascular cause. A stroke specialist determined whether a stroke has occurred and determined the stroke severity using the National Institutes of Health Stroke Scale transient ischemic attack/stroke questionnaire. Available neuroimaging studies were considered to support the clinical impression and to determine if there was a demonstrable lesion compatible with an acute stroke. Strokes were classified as ischemic, hemorrhagic, or unknown. Four criteria had to be fulfilled to diagnose stroke:
	1. Rapid onset of a focal/global neurologic deficit with at least 1 of the following: change in level of consciousness, hemiplegia, hemiparesis, numbness or sensory loss affecting 1 side of the body, dysphasia/aphasia, hemianopia, amaurosis fugax, and other new neurologic sign(s)/symptom(s) consistent with stroke
	2. Duration of a focal/global neurologic deficit $\geq$24 h or <24 h if any of the following conditions existed:
	  i. At least 1 of the following therapeutic interventions:
	    a. Pharmacologic (ie, thrombolytic drug administration)
	    b. Nonpharmacologic (ie, neurointerventional procedure, such as intracranial angioplasty)
	  ii. Available brain imaging clearly documents a new hemorrhage or infarct
	  iii. The neurologic deficit results in death

(continued on next page)

Endpoint	Definition
	3. No other readily identifiable nonstroke cause for the clinical presentation
	4. Confirmation of the diagnosis by a neurology or neurosurgical specialist and at least 1 of the following:
	a. Brain imaging procedure (at least 2 of the following):
	• Computed tomography scan
	• Magnetic resonance imaging scan
	• Cerebral vessel angiography
	b. Lumbar puncture (ie, spinal fluid analysis diagnostic of intracranial hemorrhage)
	All strokes with stroke disability of modified Rankin Scale score ≥1 (increase from baseline assessment) were included in the primary endpoint.

Adapted from Kappetein AP, Serruys PW, Sabik JF, et al. Design and rationale for a randomised comparison of everolimus-eluting stents and coronary artery bypass graft surgery in selected patients with left main coronary artery disease: the EXCEL trial. EuroIntervention 2016;12:861–872; with permission.

0.88; $P = .008$), which was driven by fewer procedural MIs (5.9% vs 3.6%, respectively; HR 0.61; 95% CI, 0.40–0.93; $P = .02$). Definite stent thrombosis or symptomatic graft failure was markedly less frequent in the PCI arm (HR 0.27; 95% CI, 0.08–0.97; $P = .03$). There also was a markedly lower incidence of major periprocedural adverse events within 30 days after PCI compared with CABG, including major bleeding, arrhythmias, prolonged intubation, acute kidney injury, and more (total 12.4% vs 44.0%, respectively; relative risk [RR] 0.28; 95% CI, 0.24–0.34; $P<.001$).[26] At 3 years, there also was no significant difference in the composite endpoint of death, MI, stroke, or ischemia-driven revascularization after PCI compared with CABG (23.1% vs 19.1%, respectively; HR 1.18; 95% CI, 0.97–1.45; $P = .10$), although repeat revascularization (TLR, TVR, and non-TVR) was more common after PCI.

In 2019, the final 5-year outcomes of EXCEL were published.[27] Again, there was no significant difference in the rates of the primary endpoint between PCI and CABG (22.0% vs 19.2%, respectively; odds ratio [OR] 1.19; 95% CI, 0.95–1.50; $P = .13$) (Fig. 1). All-cause death was more frequent in the PCI group (13.0% vs 9.9%, respectively; OR 1.38%; 95% CI, 1.03–1.85), which was driven by greater non-cardiovascular death (OR 1.47; 95% CI, 0.97–2.23; mainly due to an excess number of deaths adjudicated as due to sepsis and cancer occurring between 1 year and 5 years after treatment). There were no differences between PCI and CABG with regard to definite cardiovascular death (5.0% and 4.5%, respectively;

OR 1.13; 95% CI, 0.73–1.74) and MI (10.6% and 9.1%, respectively; OR 1.14; 95% CI, 0.84–1.55). The incidence of stroke also was nonsignificantly different (2.9% and 3.7%, respectively; OR 0.78; 95% CI, 0.46–1.31), although all cerebrovascular events were less with PCI compared with CABG (3.3% vs 5.2%, respectively; OR 0.61; 95% CI, 0.38–0.99). Ischemia-driven revascularization was more frequent after PCI (16.9% vs 10.0%, respectively; OR 1.84; 95% CI, 1.39–2.44). Subgroup analysis did not identify significant interactions (Fig. 2).

Due to the nonproportional hazards at different time points during the 5-year follow-up, piecewise hazard model analysis was used, splitting follow-up time in 3 different periods, representing periprocedural (0–30 days), midterm (30 days–1 year), and long-term (1–5 years) risks,[28] thus calculating HRs separately within each segment (Fig. 3). During the first 30 days after revascularization, PCI was associated with a lower risk of the primary endpoint (HR 0.61; 95% CI, 0.42–0.88), which was driven by a lower incidence of (procedural) MI (HR 0.63; 95% CI, 0.42–0.94). Between 30 days and 1 year, the primary endpoint rates between PCI and CABG were similar (HR 1.07; 95% CI, 0.68–1.70), as were each of its individual components. Between 1 year and 5 years, the risk for the primary endpoint was higher in the PCI arm (HR 1.61; 95% CI, 1.23–2.12), which was driven by numerically more deaths and MIs. These data indicate that the early benefit of PCI gradually was eroded over time by an increased postprocedural risk. Ischemia-driven revascularization also was more likely in PCI patients within 5 years,

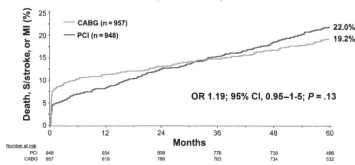

Primary Endpoint
All-cause Death, S/stroke, or MI at 5 Y

OR 1.19; 95% CI, 0.95–1-5; *P* = .13

Fig. 1. Time-to-first-event curves for the EXCEL trial primary endpoint through 5-year follow-up. (*Adapted from* Stone GW, Kappetein AP, Sabik JF, et al. Five-year outcomes after PCI or CABG for left main coronary disease. N. Engl. J. Med. 2019;381:1820–1830; with permission.)

with an absolute difference of approximately 7%. The mean time free from a primary endpoint event during the 5 year follow-up period was 5.2 days (95% CI, −46.1 to 56.5 days) longer after PCI compared with CABG, representing nearly identical long-term freedom from the burden of these major adverse events.[27]

KEY EVALUATION OF XIENCE VERSUS CORONARY ARTERY BYPASS SURGERY FOR EFFECTIVENESS OF LEFT MAIN REVASCULARIZATION TRIAL SUBSTUDIES

EXCEL has provided insightful data on key subgroups and secondary endpoints, which have the potential to inform clinical decision making and the design of further prospective studies.

A substudy[29] provided data on the incidence of new-onset atrial fibrillation (NOAF) after LM CAD revascularization. NOAF developed at a mean of 2.7 days ± 2.5 days after revascularization in 18.0% of CABG patients versus 0.1% of PCI patients (*P*<.0001). Patients who developed NOAF had longer hospital stays, were more likely to be discharged on anticoagulant therapy, and had an increased 30-day rate of Thrombolysis In Myocardial Infarction major or minor bleeding (14.2% vs 5.5%, respectively; *P*<.0001). By multivariable analysis, NOAF after CABG was an independent predictor of 3-year stroke (6.6% vs 2.4%, respectively; adjusted HR 4.19; 95% CI, 1.74–10.11; *P* = .001), death (11.4% vs 4.3%, respectively; adjusted HR 3.02; 95% CI, 1.60–5.70; *P* = .0006), and the primary composite endpoint of death, MI, or stroke (22.6% vs 12.8%, respectively; adjusted HR 2.13; 95% CI, 1.39–3.25; *P* = .0004).

Analysis of 10 pre-specified subgroups
All-cause Death, S/stroke, or MI at 5 Y

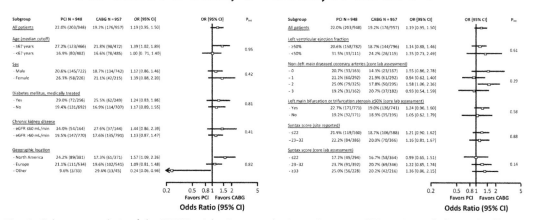

Fig. 2. Subgroup analysis of the EXCEL trial primary endpoint at 5 years. eGFR, estimated glomerular filtration rate. (*Adapted from* Stone GW, Kappetein AP, Sabik JF, et al. Five-year outcomes after PCI or CABG for left main coronary disease. N. Engl. J. Med. 2019;381:1820–1830; with permission.)

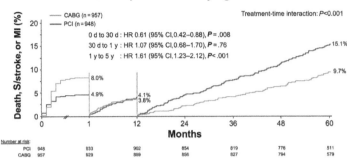

Fig. 3. Piecewise hazard analysis of the EXCEL trial primary endpoint through 5-year follow-up. (*Adapted from* Stone GW, Kappetein AP, Sabik JF, et al. Five-year outcomes after PCI or CABG for left main coronary disease. N. Engl. J. Med. 2019;381:1820–1830; with permission.)

A subanalysis focusing on diabetics (29%) versus nondiabetics (71%)[30] showed that the 3-year primary endpoint was more frequent in diabetic patients (20.0% vs 12.9%, respectively; HR 1.60; 95% CI, 1.26–2.04; $P<.001$). There was no interaction for treatment effect, however, with PCI versus CABG in diabetics (20.7% vs 19.3%, respectively; HR 1.03; 95% CI, 0.71–1.50; $P = .87$) and nondiabetics (12.9% vs 12.9%, respectively; HR 0.98; 95% CI, 0.73–1.32; $P = .89$) (P for interaction = 0.82). All-cause death at 3 years occurred in 13.6% of PCI and 8.0% of CABG patients ($P = .046$), although no significant interaction was present between diabetes status and treatment of all-cause death ($P = .22$), MI ($P = .99$), or stroke ($P = .17$). Ischemia-driven revascularization was more common with PCI both in diabetics (16.9% vs 8.7%, respectively; $P = .008$) and nondiabetics (11.0% vs 7.0%, respectively; $P = .01$), with no interaction between subgroups ($P = .51$). On the basis of this study, diabetes did not seem to be a major risk factor dictating whether LM-CAD patients should undergo PCI versus CABG.

Another study evaluated the impact of chronic kidney disease (CKD), defined as an estimated glomerular filtration rate less than 60 mL/min/1.73 m^2.[31] CKD was present in 19.3% of patients. Patients with CKD had higher rates of the primary endpoint at 3 years (20.8% vs 13.5%, respectively; HR 1.60; 95% CI, 1.22–2.09; $P = .0005$). Acute renal failure (a serum creatinine increase ≥5.0 mg/dL from baseline or new need for dialysis) within 30 days occurred more commonly in patients with CKD (5.0% vs 0.8%, respectively; $P<.0001$) and was strongly associated with the 3-year risk of the primary endpoint (50.7% vs 14.4%, respectively; HR 4.59; 95% CI, 2.73–7.73; $P<.0001$). Acute renal failure

occurred less frequently after revascularization with PCI compared with CABG both in patients with (2.3% vs 7.7%, respectively; HR 0.28; 95% CI, 0.09–0.87) and without (0.3% vs 1.3%, respectively; HR 0.20; 95% CI, 0.04–0.90) CKD (P for interaction = 0.71). There were no significant differences in the rates of the primary composite endpoint after PCI and CABG in patients with (23.4% vs 18.1%, respectively; HR 1.25; 95% CI, 0.79–1.98) and without (13.4% vs 13.5%, respectively; HR 0.97; 95% CI, 0.73–1.27) CKD (P for interaction = 0.38).

A QOL analysis from EXCEL[32] showed that both revascularization modalities were associated with significant improvements in QOL from baseline to 36 months. At 30 days, PCI was associated with better QOL, less dyspnea, and greater improvement in angina relief than CABG. Depression also was less after PCI compared with CABG. By 12 months, however, these differences largely were attenuated, and by 36 months there were no significant differences in QOL between PCI and CABG.

Another substudy explored the impact of repeat revascularization on mortality in the EXCEL trial.[33] Repeat revascularization was required more commonly after PCI compared with CABG at 3-year follow-up (12.9% vs 7.6%, respectively; HR 1.73; 95% CI, 1.28–2.33; $P = .0003$). Need for repeat revascularization (with either PCI or CABG) was independently associated with increased risk for all-cause mortality (adjusted HR 2.05; 95% CI, 1.13–3.70; $P = .02$) and cardiovascular mortality (adjusted HR 4.22; 95% CI, 2.10–8.48; $P<.0001$) consistently after both PCI and CABG (P for interaction = 0.85 for both). Although TVR and TLR both were associated with an increased risk for mortality, target vessel non-TLR and non-TVR were not.

Finally, another report looked at the impact of procedural MI on mortality in the EXCEL trial.[34] As detailed in Table 1, to minimize event ascertainment bias between the procedures, procedural MI was defined using identical definitions and biomarker thresholds for PCI and CABG (peak CK-MB elevation >10× the upper reference limit [URL] within 72 h postprocedure, or >5× URL with new Q-waves, angiographic vessel occlusion, or loss of myocardium on imaging). Procedural MI occurred in 3.6% versus 6.1%, respectively, of patients in the PCI versus CABG groups (OR 0.61; 95% CI, 0.40–0.93; $P = .02$). Procedural MI was associated with cardiovascular death (adjusted HR 2.63; 95% CI, 1.19–5.81; $P = .02$) and all-cause death (adjusted HR 2.28; 95% CI, 1.22–4.29; $P = .01$) at 3-year follow-up. The effect of procedural MI was consistent after both PCI and CABG for cardiovascular death (P for interaction = 0.56) and all-cause death (P for interaction = 0.59). Peak postprocedure CK-MB greater than or equal to 10× URL strongly predicted mortality, whereas lesser degrees of myonecrosis were not associated with prognosis.

EVALUATION OF XIENCE VERSUS CORONARY ARTERY BYPASS SURGERY FOR EFFECTIVENESS OF LEFT MAIN REVASCULARIZATION TRIAL CONTROVERSIES

As discussed previously, primary endpoint analysis of EXCEL did not identify differences in the rates of the primary endpoint at 3-year follow-up, and extended follow-up at 5 years highlighted a complex pattern of nonproportional hazards, in which PCI exhibited better outcomes at 30 days (mainly related to a lower risk for procedural MI), equipoise between PCI and CABG between 30 days and 1 year, and lower risk of the primary endpoint with CABG between 1 year and 5 years (which was driven by fewer late noncardiovascular deaths and MIs).

Two study findings from EXCEL deserve special consideration. First, was the increased risk of death observed with PCI truly indicative of worse outcomes attributable to LM percutaneous revascularization? As discussed previously, cardiovascular mortality was not different between PCI and CABG (consistent with the overall similar rates of MI between the 2 revascularization modalities). Rather, the observed differences in all-cause death were driven mainly by noncardiovascular mortality secondary to late sepsis and cancer, which are of uncertain biologic plausibility. Moreover, approximately 35 secondary endpoints (for

which the trial was not powered) were examined, raising concern for a chance finding (P values were not adjusted for multiple comparisons).

To better assess low-frequency nonpowered endpoints, examining the totality of the evidence from other high-quality RCTs is useful. Two recent meta-analyses did not observe a difference in all-cause mortality between PCI and CABG in patients undergoing LM revascularization. Head and colleagues[35] performed an individual patient data pooled analysis of 11 RCTs, including patients undergoing PCI versus CABG for multivessel CAD or LM stenosis (n = 11,518 patients). Although PCI was associated with higher risk for 5-year all-cause mortality (11.2% vs 9.2%, respectively; HR 1.20; 95% CI, 1.06–1.37; $P = .0038$), this finding was driven by differences in patients with multivessel CAD and diabetes. Patients with multivessel CAD without diabetes and those with LM disease (with or without diabetes) had similar mortality rates (LM cohort PCI vs CABG at 5 years: 10.7% vs 10.5%, respectively; HR 1.07%; 95% 0.87–1.33; $P = .52$). A more recent meta-analysis that focused on patients undergoing LM revascularization[36] included 5 RCTs for a total of 4612 patients. At a mean follow-up of 67.1 months, there were no differences between PCI and CABG for the risk of all-cause death (RR 1.03; 95% CI, 0.81–1.32; $P = .779$) or cardiac death (RR 1.03; 95% CI, 0.79–1.34; $P = .817$) (Fig. 4). There also were no significant differences in the long-term risks of stroke (RR 0.74; 95% CI, 0.35–1.50; $P = .400$) or MI (RR 1.22; 95% CI, 0.96–1.56; $P = .110$). PCI was associated with an increased risk of unplanned revascularization (RR 1.73; 95% CI, 1.49–2.02; $P<.001$). Ten-year follow-up from the SYNTAX trial also showed similar rates of death between PCI and CABG (26% vs 28%, respectively; HR 0.9; 95% CI, 0.68–1.20; $P = .47$).[14] In summary, the totality of evidence supports the notion that PCI and CABG are associated with similar rates of all-cause death at long-term follow-up, with the EXCEL trial finding of a borderline higher mortality in patients undergoing PCI most likely due to play of chance (mainly driven by noncardiovascular mortality).

The second controversial finding related to the differences in the risk for MI after PCI versus CABG during follow-up. Compared with PCI, CABG resulted in a higher rate of procedural MI in the early postoperative period but lower rates of MI between 1 year and 5 years (likely due to fewer spontaneous MIs arising from diseased atherosclerotic segments proximal to graft anastomoses compared with untreated nonstented

A

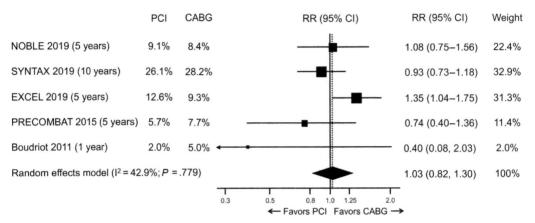

Meta-analysis
Long-Term All-Cause Death (n = 4,595)

B

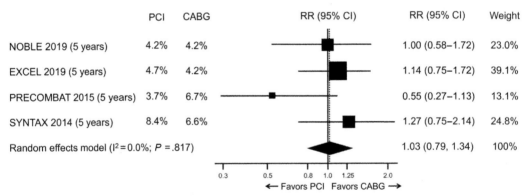

Meta-analysis
Long-Term Cardiac Death (n = 4,394)

Fig. 4. Meta-analysis for long-term (A) all-cause death and (B) cardiac death in RCTs comparing PCI with DESs versus CABG for LM revascularization. (*Adapted from* Ahmad Y, Howard JP, Arnold AD, et al. Mortality after drug-eluting stents vs. coronary artery bypass grafting for left main coronary artery disease: a meta-analysis of randomized controlled trials. Eur. Heart J. 2020; with permission.)

segments). Thus, the primary endpoint was dependent on the definitions of MI in these 2 periods, and some have wondered why the specific protocol definition of MI was chosen rather than the Universal Definition definition of MI (UDMI).[37] The protocol procedural MI definition in EXCEL was similar to the Society for Cardiovascular Angiography and Interventions definition of a clinically relevant MI[38] and required a marked elevation of CK-MB (>10× URL or >5× with ancillary ECG/angiographic/imaging ischemic findings) to diagnose procedural MIs, whereas lower and more sensitive elevations (troponin or CK-MB >1× URL) were utilized to adjudicate spontaneous MI. EXCEL was designed and led by a large academic physician group consisting

of an equal number of cardiac surgeons and interventionalists. A large biomarker increase was required for the procedural MI definition because in most prior studies only such large indicators of myonecrosis were correlated with subsequent death.[39-41] In contrast, for spontaneous MI, even small elevations of troponin have been strongly associated with high rates of death during follow-up.[42] As discussed previously, data from EXCEL[34] demonstrated that only large procedural MIs (eg, peak postprocedure CK-MB ≥10× URL[34,41]) were associated with mortality, whereas lesser degrees of myonecrosis were not.

In the EXCEL trial, procedural MI according to the Third UDMI was listed as a secondary endpoint[37] but has not yet been reported, which has raised concerns by some critics.[43] The UDMI utilizes cardiac troponin as its preferred biomarker with different biomarker thresholds after PCI and CABG and requires additional supporting data, such as clinical, ECG, angiographic, or imaging findings, which also differ after PCI and CABG, potentially introducing ascertainment bias (Table 2). For example, troponin levels must be normal at baseline to diagnose post-CABG MI but not to adjudicate post-PCI MI; symptoms are a criterion for post-PCI MI but not for post-CABG MI; and ischemic ECG changes are required to diagnose post-PCI MI whereas Q-waves are needed to adjudicate post-CABG MI. In addition, the biomarker cutoffs in the UDMI ($>5\times$ URL for PCI and $>10\times$ URL for CABG) admittedly were arbitrarily selected and show poor correlation with clinical outcomes.[38] For all these reasons, the surgeons and interventional cardiologists who designed EXCEL selected the more rigorous and specific protocol definition for procedural MI rather than the Third UDMI. Moreover, whereas CK-MB assessments at baseline and postprocedure were mandatory in EXCEL, troponin elevations were optional and were drawn in fewer than 50% of patients. Thus, any reporting of the Third UDMI either needs to be limited to this subpopulation (representing a biased cohort) or include a mix of biomarkers, which have markedly differing sensitivities. Despite these limitations, the EXCEL investigators have committed to report alternative rates of procedural MI and their implications (correlation with cardiovascular and all-cause death) in 2020.

EVALUATION OF XIENCE VERSUS CORONARY ARTERY BYPASS SURGERY FOR EFFECTIVENESS OF LEFT MAIN REVASCULARIZATION TRIAL IN PERSPECTIVE AND CURRENT RECOMMENDATIONS

The EXCEL trial represents the largest contemporary RCT assessing the impact of revascularization strategies for LM disease using a clinically meaningful primary endpoint. In summary, key study findings are (1) no significant differences were observed for the primary endpoint of all-cause death, stroke, or MI at either 3-year or 5-year follow-up between PCI and CABG; (2) in the early postoperative period, CABG was associated with higher risk of the primary endpoint, driven by greater rates of large

Table 2
Procedural myocardial infarction definitions per the Third Universal Definition of Myocardial Infarction

Type 4a (post-PCI)	MI is defined arbitrarily by elevation of troponin $>5 \times$ 99th percentile URL in patients with normal baseline values or rise $>20\%$ if the baseline values are elevated and stable or falling, plus 1 of the following: 1. Symptoms suggestive of myocardial ischemia 2. New ischemic ECG changes or new left bundle branch block 3. Angiographic loss of patency of a major coronary artery or side branch or persistent slow or no reflow of embolization 4. Imaging demonstration of new loss of viable myocardium or new regional wall motion abnormality
Type 5 (post-CABG)	MI is arbitrarily defined by elevation of biomarker $>10 \times$ 99th percentile URL in patients with normal baseline values, plus 1 of the following: 1. New Q-waves or new left bundle branch block 2. Angiographic documented new graft or new native coronary artery occlusion 3. Imaging demonstration of new loss of viable myocardium or new regional wall motion abnormality
Issues	Ascertainment and other biases • Must have normal biomarker levels for post-CABG MI but not for post-PCI MI • Symptoms are a criteria post-PCI but not post-CABG • Ischemic ECG changes required post-PCI vs Q-waves post-CABG • Angiography is performed in 100% of PCI patients vs rarely after CABG

Adapted from Thygesen K, Alpert JS, Jaffe AS, et al. Third universal definition of myocardial infarction. Eur. Heart J. 2012;33:2551–67; with permission.

procedural MI, often due to symptomatic graft occlusion; (3) CABG also resulted in a marked increase in periprocedural rates of major bleeding and transfusions, NOAF requiring cardioversion or anticoagulation, acute kidney injury, sepsis, prolonged intubation and sternal wound dehiscence, and other periprocedural complications; (4) PCI and CABG provided similar outcomes between 1 month and 1 year after LM revascularization; (5) PCI was associated with a higher incidence of the primary endpoint between 1 year and 5 years, which was driven by greater rates of spontaneous MI and all-cause (mainly noncardiovascular) deaths; (6) PCI also was associated with greater rates of repeat revascularization during long-term follow-up, although with lower rates of all cerebrovascular events; and (7) QOL improvement and angina relief initially were better within 30 days after PCI but similar after both PCI and CABG during long-term follow-up.

Although no US guidelines have been published after the EXCEL trial results were published, the 2018 European guidelines on myocardial revascularization[6] include recommendations based on the EXCEL trial 3-year results.[26] This document states that PCI is an appropriate alternative to CABG in patients with LM disease and low to intermediate anatomic complexity (SYNTAX score ≤32), resulting in a class I recommendation for low anatomic complexity (SYNTAX score ≤22) and a class IIa recommendation for intermediate anatomic complexity (SYNTAX score >22–32) (because the 5-year follow-up of EXCEL and NOBLE had not yet been reported). Among patients with LM disease and high anatomic complexity (SYNTAX score >32), the number of patients studied in RCTs was low due to exclusion criteria; as such, the risk estimates and CIs are imprecise but suggest a trend toward better survival with CABG.[35] Therefore, PCI in this setting has a class III recommendation (contraindication). In a large South Korean registry[44] (n = 1580), PCI in patients with high SYNTAX scores was associated with a higher risk for death (adjusted HR 1.39; 95% CI, 1.00–1.92; $P = .048$) and a trend toward a higher risk of a composite of death, Q-wave MI, and stroke (adjusted HR 1.27; 95% CI, 0.94–1.74; $P = .123$) at 10-year follow-up compared with CABG. A major limitation of this study, however, is that PCI was performed with BMSs or first-generation DESs. In the EXCEL trial, the primary endpoint results after PCI and CABG were consistent in patients with low, intermediate, and high SYNTAX scores, as assessed by the angiographic core laboratory. Therefore, at present, there is no solid evidence demonstrating a higher mortality with state-of-the-art PCI using second-generation DESs in patients with LM disease, compared with CABG, across any stratum of anatomic complexity, although in general CABG is preferred in patients with highly complex coronary anatomy and acceptable surgical risk.

In summary, PCI and CABG are 2 very different procedures. Although the overall long-term rates of death, MI, and stroke will be similar after both for many patients with LM-CAD, the relative risk of early and late adverse events with each procedure varies. In addition, a substantial proportion of patients has specific clinical or anatomic features either strongly indicating one or contraindicating the other procedure (eg, multiple chronic total occlusions leading to a clear choice for CABG or patient frailty or severe lung disease leading to a clear choice for PCI). The risks and benefits of each procedure should be discussed with each patient, taking into account each individual's specific clinical and anatomic risk factors, with patient preferences strongly considered when deciding between PCI and CABG.

DISCLOSURE

Dr L. Azzalini has received honoraria from Abbott Vascular, Guerbet, Terumo, and Sahajanand Medical Technologies and research support from ACIST Medical Systems, Guerbet, and Terumo. Dr G.W. Stone has received speaker or other honoraria from Cook, Terumo, QOOL Therapeutics, and Orchestra Biomed; served as a consultant to Valfix, TherOx, Vascular Dynamics, Robocath, HeartFlow, Gore, Ablative Solutions, Miracor, Neovasc, V-Wave, Abiomed, Ancora, MAIA Pharmaceuticals, Vectorious, Reva, and Matrizyme; and received equity/options from Ancora, Qool Therapeutics, Cagent, Applied Therapeutics, Biostar family of funds, SpectraWave, Orchestra Biomed, Aria, Cardiac Success, MedFocus family of funds, and Valfix.

REFERENCES

1. Ragosta M, Dee S, Sarembock IJ, et al. Prevalence of unfavorable angiographic characteristics for percutaneous intervention in patients with unprotected left main coronary artery disease. Catheter Cardiovasc Interv 2006;68:357–62.

2. D'Ascenzo F, Presutti DG, Picardi E, et al. Prevalence and non-invasive predictors of left main or three-vessel coronary disease: evidence from a collaborative international meta-analysis including 22 740 patients. Heart 2012;98:914–9.

3. Taggart DP, Kaul S, Boden WE, et al. Revascularization for unprotected left main stem coronary artery

stenosis stenting or surgery. J Am Coll Cardiol 2008;51:885–92.

4. Serruys PW, Morice MC, Kappetein AP, et al. Percutaneous coronary intervention versus coronary-artery bypass grafting for severe coronary artery disease. N Engl J Med 2009;360:327–34.

5. Levine GN, Bates ER, Blankenship JC, et al. 2011 ACCF/AHA/SCAI guideline for percutaneous coronary intervention a report of the American College of Cardiology Foundation/American Heart Association Task Force on Practice Guidelines and the Society for Cardiovascular Angiography and Interventions. Circulation 2011;124:574–651.

6. Neumann F-J, Sousa-Uva M, Ahlsson A, et al. 2018 ESC/EACTS guidelines on myocardial revascularization. Eur Heart J 2019;40:87–165.

7. Conley MJ, Ely RL, Kisslo J, et al. The prognostic spectrum of left main stenosis. Circulation 1978; 57:947–52.

8. Takaro T, Peduzzi P, Detre KM, et al. Survival in subgroups of patients with left main coronary artery disease. Veterans Administration Cooperative Study of Surgery for Coronary Arterial Occlusive Disease. Circulation 1982;66:14–22.

9. Yusuf S, Zucker D, Peduzzi P, et al. Effect of coronary artery bypass graft surgery on survival: overview of 10-year results from randomised trials by the Coronary Artery Bypass Graft Surgery Trialists Collaboration. Lancet 1994;344:563–70.

10. Chaitman BR, Fisher LD, Bourassa MG, et al. Effect of coronary bypass surgery on survival patterns in subsets of patients with left main coronary artery disease. Report of the Collaborative Study in Coronary Artery Surgery (CASS). Am J Cardiol 1981;48: 765–77.

11. Caracciolo EA, Davis KB, Sopko G, et al. Comparison of surgical and medical group survival in patients with left main equivalent coronary artery disease. Long-term CASS experience. Circulation 1995;91:2335–44.

12. Hlatky MA, Boothroyd DB, Bravata DM, et al. Coronary artery bypass surgery compared with percutaneous coronary interventions for multivessel disease: a collaborative analysis of individual patient data from ten randomised trials. Lancet 2009;373:1190–7.

13. Byrne RA, Joner M, Kastrati A. Stent thrombosis and restenosis: what have we learned and where are we going? The Andreas Grüntzig Lecture ESC 2014. Eur Heart J 2015;36:3320–31.

14. Thuijs DJFM, Kappetein AP, Serruys PW, et al. Percutaneous coronary intervention versus coronary artery bypass grafting in patients with three-vessel or left main coronary artery disease: 10-year follow-up of the multicentre randomised controlled SYNTAX trial. Lancet 2019;394:1325–34.

15. Ahn J-M, Roh J-H, Kim Y-H, et al. Randomized trial of stents versus bypass surgery for left main coronary artery disease: 5-year outcomes of the PRECOMBAT study. J Am Coll Cardiol 2015;65:2198–206.

16. Mäkikallio T, Holm NR, Lindsay M, et al. Percutaneous coronary angioplasty versus coronary artery bypass grafting in treatment of unprotected left main stenosis (NOBLE): a prospective, randomised, open-label, non-inferiority trial. Lancet 2016;388: 2743–52.

17. Armstrong PW, Westerhout CM. Composite end points in clinical research: a time for reappraisal. Circulation 2017;135:2299–307.

18. Rittger H, Frosch B, Vitali-Serdoz L, et al. Differences of patients' perceptions for elective diagnostic coronary angiography and percutaneous coronary intervention in stable coronary artery disease between elderly and younger patients. Clin Interv Aging 2018;13:1935–43.

19. Kappetein AP, Serruys PW, Sabik JF, et al. Design and rationale for a randomised comparison of everolimus-eluting stents and coronary artery bypass graft surgery in selected patients with left main coronary artery disease: the EXCEL trial. EuroIntervention 2016;12:861–72.

20. Palmerini T, Benedetto U, Biondi-Zoccai G, et al. Long-term safety of drug-eluting and bare-metal stents: evidence from a comprehensive network meta-analysis. J Am Coll Cardiol 2015;65:2496–507.

21. Dangas GD, Serruys PW, Kereiakes DJ, et al. Meta-analysis of everolimus-eluting versus paclitaxel-eluting stents in coronary artery disease: final 3-year results of the SPIRIT clinical trials program (Clinical Evaluation of the Xience V Everolimus Eluting Coronary Stent System in the Treatment of Patients With De Novo Native Coronary Artery Lesions). JACC Cardiovasc Interv 2013;6:914–22.

22. Toyota T, Shiomi H, Morimoto T, et al. Meta-analysis of long-term clinical outcomes of everolimus-eluting stents. Am J Cardiol 2015;116:187–94.

23. Head SJ, Börgermann J, Osnabrugge RLJ, et al. Coronary artery bypass grafting: Part 2–optimizing outcomes and future prospects. Eur Heart J 2013; 34:2873–86.

24. Kieser TM, Head SJ, Kappetein AP. Arterial grafting and complete revascularization: challenge or compromise? Curr Opin Cardiol 2013;28:646–53.

25. Samadashvili Z, Sundt TM 3rd, Wechsler A, et al. Multiple versus single arterial coronary bypass graft surgery for multivessel disease. J Am Coll Cardiol 2019;74:1275–85.

26. Stone GW, Sabik JF, Serruys PW, et al. Everolimus-eluting stents or bypass surgery for left main coronary artery disease. N Engl J Med 2016;375: 2223–35.

27. Stone GW, Kappetein AP, Sabik JF, et al. Five-year outcomes after PCI or CABG for left main coronary disease. N Engl J Med 2019;381:1820–30.

28. Gregson J, Sharples L, Stone GW, et al. Nonproportional hazards for time-to-event outcomes in clinical trials: JACC review topic of the week. J Am Coll Cardiol 2019;74:2102–12.

29. Kosmidou I, Chen S, Kappetein AP, et al. New-onset atrial fibrillation after PCI or CABG for left main disease: the EXCEL trial. J Am Coll Cardiol 2018;71:739–48.

30. Milojevic M, Serruys PW, Sabik JF 3rd, et al. Bypass surgery or stenting for left main coronary artery disease in patients with diabetes. J Am Coll Cardiol 2019;73:1616–28.

31. Giustino G, Mehran R, Serruys PW, et al. Left main revascularization with PCI or CABG in patients with chronic kidney disease: EXCEL trial. J Am Coll Cardiol 2018;72:754–65.

32. Baron SJ, Chinnakondepalli K, Magnuson EA, et al. Quality-of-life after everolimus-eluting stents or bypass surgery for left-main disease: results from the EXCEL trial. J Am Coll Cardiol 2017;70: 3113–22.

33. Giustino G, Serruys PW, Sabik JF 3rd, et al. Mortality after repeat revascularization following PCI or CABG for left main disease: the EXCEL Trial. JACC Cardiovasc Interv 2020;13:375–87.

34. Ben-Yehuda O, Chen S, Redfors B, et al. Impact of large periprocedural myocardial infarction on mortality after percutaneous coronary intervention and coronary artery bypass grafting for left main disease: an analysis from the EXCEL trial. Eur Heart J 2019;40:1930–41.

35. Head SJ, Milojevic M, Daemen J, et al. Mortality after coronary artery bypass grafting versus percutaneous coronary intervention with stenting for coronary artery disease: a pooled analysis of individual patient data. Lancet 2018;391:939–48.

36. Ahmad Y, Howard JP, Arnold AD, et al. Mortality after drug-eluting stents vs. coronary artery bypass grafting for left main coronary artery disease: a meta-analysis of randomized controlled trials. Eur Heart J 2020. https://doi.org/10.1093/eurheartj/ehaa135.

37. Thygesen K, Alpert JS, Jaffe AS, et al. Third universal definition of myocardial infarction. Eur Heart J 2012;33:2551–67.

38. Moussa ID, Klein LW, Shah B, et al. Consideration of a new definition of clinically relevant myocardial infarction after coronary revascularization: an expert consensus document from the Society for Cardiovascular Angiography and Interventions (SCAI). J Am Coll Cardiol 2013;62:1563–70.

39. Lindsey JB, Kennedy KF, Stolker JM, et al. Prognostic implications of creatine kinase-MB elevation after percutaneous coronary intervention: results from the Evaluation of Drug-Eluting Stents and Ischemic Events (EVENT) registry. Circ Cardiovasc Interv 2011;4:474–80.

40. Stone GW, Mehran R, Dangas G, et al. Differential impact on survival of electrocardiographic Q-wave versus enzymatic myocardial infarction after percutaneous intervention: a device-specific analysis of 7147 patients. Circulation 2001;104:642–7.

41. Brener SJ, Ellis SG, Schneider J, et al. Frequency and long-term impact of myonecrosis after coronary stenting. Eur Heart J 2002;23:869–76.

42. Prasad A, Rihal CS, Lennon RJ, et al. Significance of periprocedural myonecrosis on outcomes after percutaneous coronary intervention: an analysis of preintervention and postintervention troponin T levels in 5487 patients. Circ Cardiovasc Interv 2008;1:10–9.

43. O'Riordan M. EXCEL investigators respond to data suppression claims as debate erupts online. tctmd.com. 2019. Available at: https://www.tctmd.com/news/excel-investigators-respond-data-suppression-claims-debate-erupts-online. Accessed June 25, 2020.

44. Yoon Y-H, Ahn J-M, Kang D-Y, et al. Impact of SYNTAX score on 10-year outcomes after revascularization for left main coronary artery disease. JACC Cardiovasc Interv 2020;13:361–71.

Complete or Incomplete Revascularization for ST-Segment Elevation Myocardial Infarction

The PRAMI Trial to COMPLETE

Matthias Bossard, MD[a], Shamir R. Mehta, MD, MSc, FRCPC, FESC[b],*

KEYWORDS

- Myocardial infarction • STEMI • Percutaneous coronary intervention • Primary PCI
- Multivessel disease • Culprit lesion • Non-infarct-related artery • Revascularization

---

KEY POINTS

- Data from randomized trials demonstrated the superiority of an approach aiming for complete revascularization versus treatment of the infarct-related lesions only among ST-segment elevation myocardial infarction (STEMI) patients with multivessel disease (MVD).
- The COMPLETE trial showed the benefit of this strategy in reducing hard outcomes of cardiovascular death or new MI, in addition to other outcomes including ischemia-driven revascularization and unstable angina.
- Meta-analyses of all randomized trials addressing this question have also demonstrated a reduction in cardiovascular mortality.
- In STEMI patients with MVD, a complete revascularization strategy with routine nonculprit lesion percutaneous coronary intervention should be considered as the standard of care.

INTRODUCTION

The management of patients presenting with ST-segment elevation myocardial infarction (STEMI) has evolved over the last three decades with improved morbidity and mortality.[1,2] Primary percutaneous coronary intervention (PCI) was a key advance contributing toward this improvement.[1,2] Despite this, some patients who present with STEMI are at increased risk of recurrent events, especially among the 30% to 50% with multivessel coronary artery disease (CAD) consisting of significant atherothrombotic lesions in locations remote from the culprit lesion.[3–7] In these patients, the question of whether to routinely revascularize nonculprit lesions with the goal of complete revascularization or whether to treat them medically with no further revascularization has been debated for many years. Although evidence derived from observational studies,[8–18] smaller randomized trials,[19–24] and several meta-analyses[4,25,26] had demonstrated routine early PCI was associated with reduced need for revascularization of the nonculprit lesion, data supporting clear reductions in hard outcomes, such as death or myocardial infarction (MI), were lacking. At least two meta-analyses suggested a possible benefit with staged nonculprit lesion PCI but until recently no single trial had demonstrated a reduction in hard clinical end points.[25,26]

---

[a] Cardiology Division, Heart Center, Luzerner Kantonsspital, Spitalstrasse 16, Luzern 6000, Switzerland;
[b] Population Health Research Institute, McMaster University, Hamilton General Hospital, Hamilton Health Sciences, 237 Barton Street East, Hamilton, Ontario L8L 2X2, Canada
* Corresponding author.
E-mail address: smehta@mcmaster.ca

Intervent Cardiol Clin 9 (2020) 433–440
https://doi.org/10.1016/j.iccl.2020.06.001
2211-7458/20/© 2020 Elsevier Inc. All rights reserved.

This review discusses the results of randomized trials comparing complete revascularization with a culprit-lesion only strategy in patients with STEMI and multivessel CAD. Moreover, we provide an overview of the existing evidence and remaining unanswered questions in this field.

THE PREVENTIVE ANGIOPLASTY IN ACUTE MYOCARDIAL INFARCTION TRIAL

The Preventive Angioplasty in Acute Myocardial Infarction (PRAMI) trial evaluated whether performing angiographically guided PCI of nonculprit lesions as part of the index primary PCI procedure reduces the combined end point of death from cardiac causes, nonfatal MI, or refractory angina.[27] In total, 465 patients with STEMI were enrolled between April 2008 through January 2013, at five centers in the United Kingdom (Table 1). During a mean follow-up of 23 months, the primary outcome of cardiac death, MI, or refractory angina was significantly lower in the multivessel PCI group versus culprit-only group (21 vs 53 events; hazard ratio [HR], 0.35; 95% confidence interval [CI], 0.21–0.58; $P<.001$). This outcome was driven mainly by a large reduction in refractory angina (16 vs 46 events; HR, 0.35; 95% CI, 0.18–0.69; $P = .002$). One limitation of this trial was that it was stopped early by the data monitoring committee for an unexpectedly large treatment effect, driven mainly by refractory angina. Refractory angina is a soft outcome in an open-label trial that is subject to bias and, together with the small absolute number of outcome events in the trial (74 in total), may have contributed to an overestimation of the true benefit.[28] Although PRAMI demonstrated promising results for the harder outcomes of cardiovascular (CV) death and MI, it was not powered or designed to reliably detect differences in these events.

THE COMPLETE VERSUS CULPRIT-LESION ONLY PRIMARY PCI TRIAL

The Complete Versus culprit-Lesion Only Primary PCI (CvLPRIT) trial enrolled 296 patients with STEMI and multivessel disease and randomized them to either PCI of the nonculprit lesion or to culprit-lesion-only PCI.[29] After 12 months of follow-up, the composite outcome of death, MI, heart failure, or repeat revascularization was lower in the multivessel PCI group compared with the culprit-only group (15 vs 31 events; HR, 0.45; 95% CI, 0.24–0.84; $P = .009$). The rates of the individual components of the

composite outcome were also numerically lower (although none were significant): death (2 vs 6), recurrent MI (2 vs 4), heart failure (4 vs 9), and repeat revascularization (7 vs 12). There was a substantial amount of patient attrition (12.5%) related to crossovers (n = 18) and loss to follow-up (n = 19).[29]

THE THIRD DANish STUDY OF OPTIMAL ACUTE TREATMENT OF PATIENTS WITH ST-SEGMENT ELEVATION MYOCARDIAL INFARCTION TRIAL

The Third DANish Study of Optimal Acute Treatment of Patients with ST-segment Elevation Myocardial Infarction (DANAMI–3–PRIMULTI) trial enrolled 627 patients presenting with STEMI and multivessel CAD and randomized them to either no further invasive treatment or to complete fractional flow reserve (FFR)-guided revascularization before discharge.[23] The primary end point of death, MI, or ischemia-driven revascularization occurred in 68 (22%) patients who had PCI of the infarct-related artery only and in 40 (13%) patients who had complete revascularization (HR, 0.56; 95% CI, 0.38–0.83; $P = .004$). This benefit was almost entirely caused by a reduction in ischemia-driven revascularization, with no difference between the groups in hard end points, including the composite of death or MI.

THE PRAGUE-13 TRIAL

The PRAGUE-13 trial randomized 214 patients with STEMI with multivessel disease to either complete revascularization with multivessel PCI or to a conservative strategy and found no significant difference in the primary composite outcome of all-cause mortality, MI, and stroke (15 vs 17 events).[24] This trial was terminated early for futility.

THE COMPARE-ACUTE TRIAL

The international Compare-Acute trial randomized 885 patients with STEMI with multivessel disease to either FFR-guided complete revascularization or treatment of the infarct artery only in a 1:2 fashion.[30] The primary outcome of a composite of death from any cause, nonfatal MI, revascularization, and stroke at 12 months occurred in 23 patients in the complete-revascularization group and in 121 patients in the infarct-artery-only group that did not undergo complete revascularization (HR, 0.35; 95% CI, 0.22–0.55; $P = .001$). This difference was driven mostly by a reduction in

Table 1
Comparison of the latest major randomized trials evaluating complete revascularization among STEMI patients

| | PRAMI[27] | CvLPRIT[29] | Major Randomized Trials (from 2013 to 2019) | | | |
			DANAMI-3–PRIMULTI[23]	PRAGUE-13[24]	Compare-Acute[30]	COMPLETE[32]
No. of countries	1	1	1	1	8	31
No. of sites	5	7	4	6	24	140
No. of patients	465	296	627	214	885	4041
Mean age (y)	62	65	63	NA	61	62
Male sex (%)	78	81	81	NA	77	80
Median follow-up (mo)	23	12	27	38	12	36
Median time from randomization to second procedure (d)	0 (same time as index procedure)	<2	2	3–40 after index procedure	0 (same time as index procedure)	1, during admission; 23, after discharge[b]
Outcomes with complete revascularization vs culprit lesion-only: % complete vs % culprit-only HR (95% CI)						
Primary end point	9 vs 23 0.35 (0.21–0.58)	10 vs 21.2 0.45 (0.24–0.84)	13 vs 22 0.56 (0.38–0.83)	16 vs 13.9 1.35 (0.66–2.74)	7.8 vs 20.5 0.35 (0.22–0.55)	7.8 vs 10.5 0.74 (0.60–0.91)[c]
All-cause mortality	5 vs 7 ns (HR NA)	1.3 vs 4.1 0.32 (0.06–1.6)	4 vs 5 1.4 (0.63–3.0)	5.7 vs 6.5 0.91 (0.3–2.7)	1.4 vs 1.7 0.80 (0.25–2.56)	4.8 vs 5.2 0.91 (0.69–1.20)
Myocardial infarction	3 vs 8.6 0.32 (0.13–0.75)	1.3 vs 2.7 0.48 (0.09–2.62)	5 vs 5 0.94 (0.47–1.9)	10.4 vs 7.4 1.71 (0.66–4.41)	2.4 vs 4.7 0.50 (0.22–1.13)	5.4 vs 7.9 0.68 (0.53–0.86)
Repeat revascularization	6.8 vs 19.9 0.30 (0.17–0.56)	4.7 vs 8.2 0.55 (0.22–1.39)	5 vs 17 0.31 (0.18–0.53)	Not published	6.1 vs 17.5 0.32 (0.20–0.54)	1.4 vs 7.9 0.18 (0.12–0.26)

Abbreviations: NA, not available in the publication; ns, nonsignificant.

[a] Illustrated are the data from the following trials: PRAMI (Preventive Angioplasty in Acute Myocardial Infarction), CvLPRIT (Complete vs Lesion-Only Primary Percutaneous Coronary Intervention [PCI] Trial), DANAMI-3–PRIMULTI (Third Danish Study of Optimal Acute Treatment of Patients with ST-Segment Elevation Myocardial Infarction [STEMI]: Primary PCI in Multivessel Disease), PRAGUE-13, Compare-Acute, and COMPLETE (Complete vs Culprit-Only Revascularization Strategies to Treat Multivessel Disease after Early PCI for STEMI).

[b] Investigators specified before randomization whether they planned to conduct the nonculprit treatment during the index hospitalization or after hospital discharge. Among the patients who underwent complete revascularization, the intended timing of the second procedure was during the index hospitalization for 1285 patients and after hospital discharge for 596 patients.

[c] The COMPLETE trial had a coprimary end point including cardiovascular death, myocardial infarction, and ischemia-driven revascularization, which was significantly lower with complete revascularization versus culprit lesion PCI only (8.9% vs 16.7%; HR, 0.51; 95% CI, 0.43–0.61).

revascularization, with no significant difference in death or new MI, although the trial was not powered to detect differences in these harder outcomes.

SEQUENTIAL META-ANALYSIS

Although none of these early trials was designed or powered to detect differences in the harder, irreversible outcomes of CV death or new MI, a trial sequential meta-analysis involving these early studies suggested that there may potentially be a benefit of complete revascularization on these outcomes, with a nominally significant reduction.[31] However, because the cumulative z curve did not cross a prespecified monitoring boundary, the evidence for reductions in hard outcomes from these trials was fragile.

THE COMPLETE TRIAL

The Complete versus Culprit-Only Revascularization Strategies to Treat Multivessel Disease after Early PCI for STEMI (COMPLETE) trial was a large-scale, multinational, comparative-effectiveness study, designed to determine whether routine, staged, angiographically guided nonculprit lesion PCI with the goal of complete revascularization reduces the risk of CV death or new MI, compared with PCI of only the culprit lesion. Following successful PCI of the culprit lesion, patients presenting with STEMI and multivessel CAD (defined as at least one additional nonculprit lesion ≥70% visual stenosis in a vessel at least 2.5 mm in diameter or 50%–70% visual stenosis with FFR <0.80) were randomized to staged, nonculprit lesion PCI with the goal of complete revascularization or to culprit lesion–only PCI, with no further revascularization of nonculprit lesions. Nonculprit lesion PCI was performed as staged procedure, either during the index hospitalization or after discharge and no later than 45 days after randomization.[32] Randomization was stratified according to the intended timing of nonculprit lesion PCI (either during or after the index hospitalization), as determined by the investigator before randomization. All coronary angiograms were reviewed by quantitative coronary angiography in a dedicated angiographic core laboratory for lesion complexity, SYNTAX score, complications, and the results of PCI. The first coprimary outcome was a composite of CV death or new MI, with the second coprimary end point comprising additionally the element of ischemia-driven revascularizations.

Overall, the trial randomized 4041 patients from 140 centers in 31 countries who had undergone primary PCI of the culprit lesion between February 2013 and March 2017.[32] The crossover rate between the two strategy groups was low (<5%). Complete revascularization, as determined by a post-PCI SYNTAX score of 0, was achieved in 90.1% of patients in the complete revascularization group. This high rate of complete revascularization allowed for a true test of the hypothesis that complete revascularization would be superior to a culprit lesion–only strategy.

At a median follow-up of 3 years, complete revascularization reduced the risk of CV death or new MI by 26% (7.8% vs 10.5%; HR, 0.74; 95% CI, 0.60–0.91; P = .004) and the risk of CV death, new MI, or ischemia-driven revascularization by 49% (8.9% vs 16.7%; HR, 0.51; 95% CI, 0.43–0.61; P<.001).[32] The benefit was driven by a significant reduction in new MI, mainly type 1 (spontaneous) MI, with a consistent directional reduction in CV death. Furthermore, the Kaplan-Meier curves for the primary end point separated early, but the benefit accrued over time, with the curves continuing to diverge over the long-term, all the way out to 5 years of follow-up (Fig. 1). Complete revascularization also substantially reduced the rates of ischemia-driven revascularization and unstable angina.

With regards to the optimal timing of nonculprit lesion PCI, the benefit of complete revascularization was similar when nonculprit PCI was performed early, at a median of 1 day during the index hospitalization (HR, 0.77; 95% CI, 0.59–1.00), or if it was performed a few weeks after hospital discharge (HR, 0.69; 95% CI, 0.49–0.97).[33] This seems attributable to the fact that the clinical benefit of complete revascularization on hard outcomes (CV death or new MI) occurs mainly over the long-term. These data suggest that most early events after STEMI are related to the size and severity of the underlying index MI or the culprit lesion primary PCI itself, whereas the benefit of PCI to the nonculprit lesion is observed mainly over the longer term.

THE COMPLETE OPTICAL COHERENCE TOMOGRAPHY SUBSTUDY

The optical coherence tomography substudy of the COMPLETE trial was designed to better understand a possible mechanistic rationale for why nonculprit lesion PCI would be of benefit in reducing hard outcomes, such as new type 1 MI. Overall 93 patients (mean age, 61 years; 83% male) underwent multivessel optical

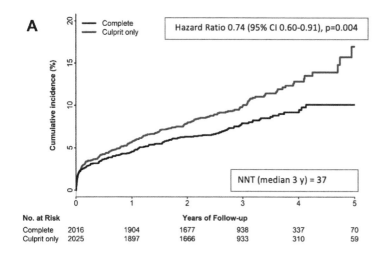

A

Hazard Ratio 0.74 (95% CI 0.60-0.91), p=0.004

— Complete
— Culprit only

NNT (median 3 y) = 37

Cumulative incidence (%)

Years of Follow-up

No. at Risk						
Complete	2016	1904	1677	938	337	70
Culprit only	2025	1897	1666	933	310	59

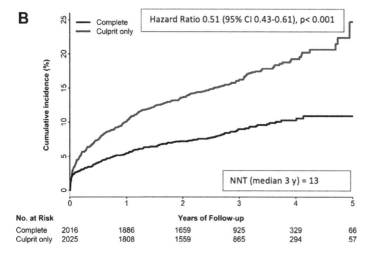

B

Hazard Ratio 0.51 (95% CI 0.43-0.61), p< 0.001

— Complete
— Culprit only

NNT (median 3 y) = 13

Cumulative incidence (%)

Years of Follow-up

No. at Risk					
Complete	2016	1886	1659	925	329	66
Culprit only	2025	1808	1559	865	294	57

Fig. 1. Incidence of the coprimary outcomes. (*A*) Cardiovascular death and new myocardial infarction and (*B*) cardiovascular death, new myocardial infarction, and ischemia driven revascularization in the COMPLETE trial. *A* and *B* illustrate Kaplan-Meier estimates of the cumulative incidence of the first coprimary outcome (death from cardiovascular causes or new myocardial infarction) and the second coprimary outcome (death from cardiovascular causes, new myocardial infarction, or ischemia-driven revascularization), respectively. NNT, number needed to treat. (*Adapted from* COMPLETE Trial – ESC 2019; Courtesy of Shamir Mehta, MD MSc.)

coherence tomography imaging and the prevalence of thin-cap fibroatheromas (TCFA) and other complex plaque features (eg, lipid content, macrophages, microvessels) was assessed in obstructive and nonobstructive nonculprit lesions among patients who were randomized to the complete revascularization arm.[34]

The prevalence of TCFA was 35.4% in obstructive lesions and 23.2% in nonobstructive lesions (*P* = .022).[34] Overall, 47.3% had an obstructive nonculprit lesion with vulnerable plaque composition, 20.4% had a nonobstructive nonculprit lesion with vulnerable plaque, and 32.3% had no nonculprit lesions with vulnerable plaque.[34] In obstructive lesions, those with TCFA were almost similar in length and lumen area to those without obstructive lesions; however, there seemed to be more lipid and other complex plaque features, namely macrophages and

cholesterol crystals (*P* for all <0.001). These data demonstrate that about one-half of nonculprit lesions contain vulnerable plaque morphology, which is more commonly found in obstructive lesions compared with nonobstructive lesions. This may be one reason why an angiographically guided nonculprit lesion PCI approach in patients with STEMI with multivessel disease was beneficial.

COLLABORATIVE META-ANALYSIS OF RANDOMIZED TRIALS

A recent collaborative meta-analysis involving 7050 patients from 10 randomized trials of complete versus culprit lesion–only PCI in patients with STEMI and multivessel CAD, found that at a mean follow-up of 29.5 months complete revascularization compared with culprit lesion–

only PCI reduced CV death (2.5% vs 3.1%; odds ratio [OR], 0.69; 95% CI, 0.48–0.99; P = .05; I^2 = 9%) and the composite of CV death or new MI (7.3% vs 10.3%; OR, 0.69; 95% CI, 0.55–0.87; P<.0002; I^2 = 6%).[35] There was no heterogeneity in the results in the trials evaluating complete revascularization performed with an FFR-guided strategy (OR, 0.78; 95% CI, 0.43–1.44) or an angiography-guided strategy (OR, 0.61; 95% CI, 0.38–0.97; P for interaction = 0.52). All-cause mortality occurred in 4.5% in the nonculprit PCI group versus 4.9% in the culprit lesion–only group (OR, 0.84; 95% CI, 0.67–1.05; P = .13; I^2 = 0%).

SAFETY OF COMPLETE REVASCULARIZATION

Possible complications of multivessel PCI in patients with STEMI include a higher risk for periprocedural complications (eg, bleeding, vascular complications, or procedure-related MI), bleeding, stroke, and contrast-induced acute kidney injury. In COMPLETE there was no significant increase in bleeding (2.9% vs 2.2%; HR, 1.33; 95% CI, 0.90–1.97), stroke (1.9% vs 1.4%; HR, 1.31; 95% CI, 0.81–2.13), or contrast-induced acute kidney injury (1.5% vs 0.9%; HR, 1.59; 95% CI, 0.89–2.84), although numerically there were more events in the complete revascularization group.

In COMPLETE, the clear benefit of complete revascularization in those patients undergoing nonculprit lesion PCI several weeks after hospital discharge is reassuring for patients with multiple comorbidities who may require additional time to recover from their index STEMI before bringing back to the cardiac catheterization laboratory for nonculprit lesion PCI. However, for most patients the staged nonculprit lesion PCI is safely performed early, including the day after the index primary PCI.

FUTURE DIRECTIONS
Which Nonculprit Lesions Should be Treated?
In several of the trials, including the COMPLETE trial, an angiographic-guided approach to achieve complete revascularization was used. Angiography-guided PCI is the most common method used to identify nonculprit lesions suitable for PCI among patients with STEMI, but may select patients who do not require PCI, resulting in unnecessary procedures, costs, and procedure-related complications. Visual estimation of stenosis severity correlates poorly with quantitative coronary angiography values assessed by angiographic core laboratories. A

physiology-guided PCI approach may overcome some of these limitations in identifying nonculprit lesions that are functionally significant. Functional significance considers not only the degree of stenosis, but also lesion length, location, and the size of the distal microcirculatory bed supplied by the coronary artery.[36] Its main benefit is in harm reduction by limiting PCI for only those lesions that are physiologically (or functionally) significant. Performing fewer PCI procedures reduces periprocedural and late events related to the PCI itself. In the context of stable CAD it has been demonstrated that an FFR-based strategy reduces the number of PCI procedures and related complications compared with an angiography-guided approach.[37] However, the clinical utility of a physiology-guided strategy to guide PCI for nonculprit lesions in STEMI remains much less clear than in stable CAD. Three randomized trials have compared FFR-guided nonculprit-lesion PCI with medical therapy alone in patients with STEMI and multivessel CAD.[19,23,30] In these trials, up to 45% of lesions identified by angiography were deferred from PCI after FFR evaluation was performed. None of these trials demonstrated reductions in the hard outcomes of CV death or new MI. By contrast, the COMPLETE trial, which used an angiography-guided strategy, showed a clear reduction in these end points. Furthermore, a recent meta-analysis comparing FFR in acute versus chronic coronary syndrome suggested that deferral of either the culprit or nonculprit lesion for PCI based on a nonischemic FFR in patients with acute coronary syndrome was associated with a higher incidence of major adverse CV events compared with patients with chronic coronary syndrome (17.6% vs 7.3%; P = .004).[38] One reason is that nonculprit lesions in STEMI are much more likely to contain vulnerable plaque morphology consisting of a TCFA and large necrotic lipid core.[39] Physiologically insignificant lesions may still harbor morphologic features (especially TCFAs) at high risk for plaque rupture or erosion leading to future CV events. The COMPLETE-2 trial will compare physiology-guided versus angiography-guided complete revascularization strategies in patients with STEMI and multivessel CAD.

SUMMARY

The question of how to manage patients with STEMI with multivessel disease has now been reliably answered. Collectively, data from randomized trials demonstrated the superiority of an approach aiming for complete revascularization versus treatment of the infarct-related lesions only. The large-scale COMPLETE trial definitively demonstrated the benefit of this strategy in reducing hard outcomes of CV death or new MI, in addition to other outcomes, including ischemia-driven revascularization and unstable angina. Meta-analyses of all randomized trials addressing this question have also demonstrated a reduction CV mortality. This approach is safe and does not significantly increase the risk for adverse event, including stroke or acute kidney injury. Based on these data, a complete revascularization strategy with routine nonculprit lesion PCI in patients with STEMI with multivessel disease should now become the standard of care. However, there is still a need for further studies and tools to identify the coronary lesions that might benefit most from PCI.

DISCLOSURE

Dr M. Bossard received consultant and speaker fees from Astra Zeneca, Amgen and Bayer. Dr S.R. Mehta reports receiving grant support from Canadian Institutes of Health Research, and research funding support from AstraZeneca and Boston Scientific.

REFERENCES

1. Gale CP, Allan V, Cattle BA, et al. Trends in hospital treatments, including revascularisation, following acute myocardial infarction, 2003-2010: a multilevel and relative survival analysis for the National Institute for Cardiovascular Outcomes Research (NICOR). Heart 2014;100(7):582–9.
2. Puymirat E, Simon T, Steg PG, et al. Association of changes in clinical characteristics and management with improvement in survival among patients with ST-elevation myocardial infarction. JAMA 2012; 308(10):998–1006.
3. Pedersen F, Butrymovich V, Kelbaek H, et al. Short- and long-term cause of death in patients treated with primary PCI for STEMI. J Am Coll Cardiol 2014;64(20):2101–8.
4. Bangalore S, Toklu B, Stone GW. Meta-analysis of culprit-only versus multivessel percutaneous coronary intervention in patients with ST-segment elevation myocardial infarction and multivessel coronary disease. Am J Cardiol 2018;121(5):529–36.
5. van der Schaaf RJ, Timmer JR, Ottervanger JP, et al. Long-term impact of multivessel disease on cause-specific mortality after ST elevation myocardial infarction treated with reperfusion therapy. Heart 2006;92(12):1760–3.
6. Sorajja P, Gersh BJ, Cox DA, et al. Impact of multivessel disease on reperfusion success and clinical outcomes in patients undergoing primary percutaneous coronary intervention for acute myocardial infarction. Eur Heart J 2007;28(14):1709–16.
7. Park DW, Clare RM, Schulte PJ, et al. Extent, location, and clinical significance of non-infarct-related coronary artery disease among patients with ST-elevation myocardial infarction. JAMA 2014; 312(19):2019–27.
8. Hannan EL, Samadashvili Z, Walford G, et al. Culprit vessel percutaneous coronary intervention versus multivessel and staged percutaneous coronary intervention for ST-segment elevation myocardial infarction patients with multivessel disease. JACC Cardiovasc Interv 2010;3(1):22–31.
9. Manari A, Varani E, Guastaroba P, et al. Long-term outcome in patients with ST segment elevation myocardial infarction and multivessel disease treated with culprit-only, immediate, or staged multivessel percutaneous revascularization strategies: insights from the REAL registry. Catheter Cardiovasc Interv 2014;84(6):912–22.
10. Barringhaus KG, Park KL, McManus DD, et al. Outcomes from patients with multi-vessel disease following primary PCI: staged PCI imparts very low mortality. Catheter Cardiovasc Interv 2011; 77(5):617–22.
11. Cavender MA, Milford-Beland S, Roe MT, et al. Prevalence, predictors, and in-hospital outcomes of non-infarct artery intervention during primary percutaneous coronary intervention for ST-segment elevation myocardial infarction (from the National Cardiovascular Data Registry). Am J Cardiol 2009;104(4):507–13.
12. Chen HC, Tsai TH, Fang HY, et al. Benefit of revascularization in non-infarct-related artery in multivessel disease patients with ST-segment elevation myocardial infarction undergoing primary percutaneous coronary intervention. Int Heart J 2010; 51(5):319–24.
13. Corpus RA, House JA, Marso SP, et al. Multivessel percutaneous coronary intervention in patients with multivessel disease and acute myocardial infarction. Am Heart J 2004;148(3):493–500.
14. Dziewierz A, Siudak Z, Rakowski T, et al. Impact of multivessel coronary artery disease and noninfarct-related artery revascularization on outcome of patients with ST-elevation myocardial infarction transferred for primary percutaneous coronary intervention (from the EUROTRANSFER Registry). Am J Cardiol 2010;106(3):342–7.
15. Kalarus Z, Lenarczyk R, Kowalczyk J, et al. Importance of complete revascularization in patients with acute myocardial infarction treated with percutaneous coronary intervention. Am Heart J 2007; 153(2):304–12.
16. Katayama N, Horiuchi K, Nakao K, et al. Does percutaneous coronary intervention in non-culprit

vessels improve the prognosis of acute myocardial infarction complicated by pump failure? J Cardiol 2005;46(1):1–8.

17. Mohamad T, Bernal JM, Kondur A, et al. Coronary revascularization strategy for ST elevation myocardial infarction with multivessel disease: experience and results at 1-year follow-up. Am J Ther 2011; 18(2):92–100.

18. Toma M, Buller CE, Westerhout CM, et al. Non-culprit coronary artery percutaneous coronary intervention during acute ST-segment elevation myocardial infarction: insights from the APEX-AMI trial. Eur Heart J 2010;31(14):1701–7.

19. Dambrink JH, Debrauwere JP, van 't Hof AW, et al. Non-culprit lesions detected during primary PCI: treat invasively or follow the guidelines? EuroIntervention 2010;5(8):968–75.

20. Di Mario C, Mara S, Flavio A, et al. Single vs multivessel treatment during primary angioplasty: results of the multicentre randomised HEpacoat for cuLPrit or multivessel stenting for Acute Myocardial Infarction (HELP AMI) Study. Int J Cardiovasc Intervent 2004;6(3-4):128–33.

21. Politi L, Sgura F, Rossi R, et al. A randomised trial of target-vessel versus multi-vessel revascularisation in ST-elevation myocardial infarction: major adverse cardiac events during long-term follow-up. Heart 2010;96(9):662–7.

22. Gershlick AH, Banning AS, Parker E, et al. Long-term follow-up of complete versus lesion-only revascularization in STEMI and multivessel disease: the CvLPRIT trial. J Am Coll Cardiol 2019;74(25):3083–94.

23. Engstrom T, Kelbaek H, Helqvist S, et al. Complete revascularisation versus treatment of the culprit lesion only in patients with ST-segment elevation myocardial infarction and multivessel disease (DANAMI-3-PRIMULTI): an open-label, randomised controlled trial. Lancet 2015;386(9994):665–71.

24. Hlinomaz O. Multivessel coronary disease diagnosed at the time of primary PCI for STEMI: complete revascularization versus conservative strategy: the PRAGUE 13 trial. EuroPCR; May 19, 2015, 2015; Paris, France.

25. Bainey KR, Mehta SR, Lai T, et al. Complete vs culprit-only revascularization for patients with multivessel disease undergoing primary percutaneous coronary intervention for ST segment elevation myocardial infarction: a systematic review and meta-analysis. Am Heart J 2014;167(1):1–14 e12.

26. Vlaar PJ, Mahmoud KD, Holmes DR Jr, et al. Culprit vessel only versus multivessel and staged percutaneous coronary intervention for multivessel disease in patients presenting with ST-segment elevation myocardial infarction: a pairwise and network meta-analysis. J Am Coll Cardiol 2011;58(7):692–703.

27. Wald DS, Morris JK, Wald NJ, et al. Randomized trial of preventive angioplasty in myocardial infarction. N Engl J Med 2013;369(12):1115–23.

28. Montori VM, Devereaux PJ, Adhikari NK, et al. Randomized trials stopped early for benefit: a systematic review. JAMA 2005;294(17):2203–9.

29. Gershlick AH, Khan JN, Kelly DJ, et al. Randomized trial of complete versus lesion-only revascularization in patients undergoing primary percutaneous coronary intervention for STEMI and multivessel disease: the CvLPRIT trial. J Am Coll Cardiol 2015;65(10):963–72.

30. Smits PC, Abdel-Wahab M, Neumann FJ, et al. Fractional flow reserve-guided multivessel angioplasty in myocardial infarction. N Engl J Med 2017;376(13):1234–44.

31. Bainey KR, Welsh RC, Toklu B, et al. Complete vs culprit-only percutaneous coronary intervention in STEMI with multivessel disease: a meta-analysis and trial sequential analysis of randomized trials. Can J Cardiol 2016;32(12):1542–51.

32. Mehta SR, Wood DA, Storey RF, et al. Complete revascularization with multivessel PCI for myocardial infarction. N Engl J Med 2019;381(15):1411–21.

33. Wood DA, Cairns JA, Wang J, et al. Timing of staged nonculprit artery revascularization in patients with ST-segment elevation myocardial infarction: COMPLETE trial. J Am Coll Cardiol 2019; 74(22):2713–23.

34. Pinilla-Echeverri N, Mehta SR, Wang J, et al. Nonculprit lesion plaque morphology in patients with ST-segment elevation myocardial infarction: results from the COMPLETE trial optical coherence tomography (OCT) substudy. Circ Cardiovasc Interv, in press.

35. Bainey KR, Engstrom T, Smits PC, et al. Complete versus culprit-lesion-only revascularization for ST-segment elevation myocardial infarction: a collaborative meta-analysis of randomized trials. JAMA Cardiol 2020. https://doi.org/10.1001/jamacardio. 2020.1251.

36. Park SJ, Kang SJ, Ahn JM, et al. Visual-functional mismatch between coronary angiography and fractional flow reserve. JACC Cardiovasc Interv 2012; 5(10):1029–36.

37. Neumann FJ, Sousa-Uva M, Ahlsson A, et al. 2018 ESC/EACTS guidelines on myocardial revascularization. Eur Heart J 2019;40(2):87–165.

38. Liou KP, Ooi S-YM, Hoole SP, et al. Fractional flow reserve in acute coronary syndrome: a meta-analysis and systematic review. Open Heart 2019; 6(1):e000934.

39. Stone GW, Maehara A, Lansky AJ, et al. A prospective natural-history study of coronary atherosclerosis. N Engl J Med 2011;364(3):226–35.

Abbreviated Dual Antiplatelet Therapy After Percutaneous Coronary Intervention in High Bleeding Risk Patients
LEADERS-FREE and ONYX ONE

Matthew J. Price, MD

KEYWORDS

- High bleeding risk • Polymer free • Durable polymer • Drug coating stent
- Zotarolimus-eluting stent • Drug-eluting stent • Antiplatelet therapy

---

KEY POINTS

- Patients can be identified as high bleeding risk (HBR) based on a set of criteria developed by the Academic Research Consortium (ARC) that predict a major bleeding rate of $\geq$4% or a risk of intracranial hemorrhage of $\geq$1% per year.
- High bleeding risk patients have not been well represented in contemporary stent trials, which require subjects to be treated with a prolonged duration of dual antiplatelet therapy.
- The LEADERS-FREE trial demonstrated that a polymer-free, drug-coated stent was safer and more effective than a bare-metal stent in patients at high bleeding risk undergoing PCI and treated with a 1-month duration of DAPT.
- The ONYX ONE trial, building on the findings of LEADERS-FREE, demonstrated that the safety and efficacy of a durable polymer zotarolimus-eluting stent were noninferior to a polymer-free drug-coated stent in HBR patients treated with 1-month of DAPT.
- Risk stratification using the ARC HBR criteria and appropriate selection of a polymer-free DCS or durable polymer zotarolimus-eluting stent may optimize clinical outcomes in patients undergoing PCI who require an abbreviated DAPT regimen.

INTRODUCTION

The optimal duration of dual antiplatelet therapy (DAPT) after percutaneous coronary intervention (PCI) with drug-eluting stents (DES) has been the focus of much discussion since early after their introduction.[1] A brief, 2- to 4-week course of aspirin and a thienopyridine after elective implantation of a bare-metal stent (BMS) became the default standard of care after this regimen was evaluated in randomized trials that observed subjects for only a short period after PCI.[2] Large prospective experiences of first-generation DES led to the adoption of a prolonged DAPT duration of at least 1 year, because unexpected episodes of late stent thrombosis were observed and were thought to be due to delayed arterial healing related in large part to an inflammatory response to durable polymers.[3] In addition to reducing the risk of late stent thrombosis, a prolonged DAPT regimen also reduces nonstent-related major adverse cardiovascular events (MACEs),[4] particularly in patients at high ischemic risk, such as

---

Division of Cardiovascular Diseases, Scripps Clinic, 9898 Genesee Avenue, AMP-200, La Jolla, CA 92037, USA
E-mail address: price.matthew@scrippshealth.org

Intervent Cardiol Clin 9 (2020) 441–449
https://doi.org/10.1016/j.iccl.2020.06.002
2211-7458/20/© 2020 Elsevier Inc. All rights reserved.

previous myocardial infarction (MI).[5,6] The risk of late stent thrombosis seems less with newer-generation stents, and Society Guidelines for DAPT duration reflect this. The 2016 American College of Cardiology (ACC)/American Heart Association (AHA) Focused Update on Duration of Dual Antiplatelet Therapy in Patients with Coronary Artery Disease recommend a DAPT duration of at least 6 months in patients with stable ischemic heart disease (SIHD) treated with DES (class I, level of evidence B); state that a DAPT duration of longer than 6 months in patients with SIHD treated with DES who have tolerated DAPT without bleeding complications and who are not at high bleeding risk (HBR) may be reasonable (class IIB, level of evidence A); and in patients with SIHD treated with DES who develop a high risk of bleeding, are at high risk of severe bleeding complication, or develop significant overt bleeding, discontinuation of $P2Y_{12}$ inhibitor therapy after 3 months may be reasonable (class IIB, level of evidence C).[7]

Many patients may not tolerate a course of DAPT beyond 1-month post-PCI because of bleeding risk. Bleeding events after PCI are associated with a subsequent mortality risk similar to an ischemic event.[8] Approximately 20% of patients aged 65 years or older receive a BMS in contemporary practice in the United States.[9] Patients receiving BMS are more likely to have a history of atrial fibrillation (AF), chronic kidney disease, bleeding risk, or an upcoming surgery.[10] In 2014, 32.1% of the AF patients presenting with acute MI and undergoing PCI in the National Cardiovascular Data Registry ACTION (Acute Coronary Treatment and Intervention Outcomes Network) Registry—Get With the Guidelines received a BMS, and 20.9% without AF received a BMS.[11] If safe, an abbreviated duration of DAPT after DES implantation in such HBR patients might provide ischemic benefit by reducing target lesion failure while reducing the risk of longer-term bleeding and its associated morbidity. However, evaluating the safety and effectiveness of DES in an HBR patient cohort is challenging, as these types of patients are typically excluded or underrepresented in clinical trials.[12] Indeed, the trials of contemporary DES—even ones that are deemed to include "all-comers"—are not generalizable to HBR patients, as patients are excluded if they are unable to take the protocol-mandated duration of DAPT, or if they are at particularly high risk for complications from DAPT (eg, previous intracranial hemorrhage, recent ischemic stroke, anemia, or thrombocytopenia).

Consensus Definition of High Bleeding Risk According to the Academic Research Consortium

The Academic Research Consortium (ARC) recently defined criteria for HBR that can act as a tool to risk-stratify patients and as a guide to appropriately design and interpret clinical trials in the HBR population.[13] Patients are deemed to be at HBR if the risk of Bleeding Academic Research Consortium (BARC) 3 or 5 bleeding is $\geq$4% or the risk of intracranial hemorrhage is $\geq$1% at 1 year. The ARC HBR criteria incorporate patient age, comorbidities, laboratory values, previous neurologic events, a history of previous bleeding, and iatrogenic factors (eg, medication or planned surgery). These criteria are listed in full in Table 1. Patients are considered to be at HBR if 1 major criterion or 2 minor criteria are met.[13]

Clinical Trials in Patients with High Bleeding Risk

Given the unmet clinical need described above, there is substantial importance for dedicated trials to examine the safety and effectiveness of DES in HBR patients treated with an abbreviated duration of DAPT. The patient populations of such trials, by necessity, will differ greatly from those in which current stents are tested. Two recent approaches have been taken to address the HBR population. The first is to leverage novel stent technology that might be particularly suitable to abbreviated DAPT. In this case, a polymer-free drug-coated stent (PF-DCS) (BioFreedom, Biosensors International, Morges, Switzerland), has been compared with the standard-of-care BMS. The improved safety and effectiveness of this approach was demonstrated in the LEADERS-FREE (Prospective Randomized Comparison of the BioFreedom Biolimus A9 Drug-Coated Stent versus the Gazelle Bare-Metal Stent in Patients at High Bleeding Risk) trial[12] and subsequently supported by the LEADERS-FREE II study (clinical trials.gov identifier NCT02843633). On the basis of these results, ONYX ONE (A Randomized Controlled Trial With Resolute Onyx in One Month Dual Antiplatelet Therapy for High-Bleeding Risk Patients) compared the newer-generation Onyx zotarolimus-eluting stent (Medtronic, Santa Rosa, CA) to the PF-DCS in an HBR population treated with 1-month DAPT,[14] and this was followed by a single-arm, observational study to provide supportive data in the North American population (clinicaltrials. gov identifier NCT03647475).

Table 1
Major and minor criteria for Academic Research Consortium-defined high bleeding risk at the time of percutaneous coronary intervention

Major	Minor
	Age $\geq$75 y
Anticipated use of long-term oral anticoagulation[a]	
Severe or end-stage CKD (eGFR <30 mL/min)	Moderate CKD (eGFR 30–59 mL/min)
Hemoglobin <11 g/dL	Hemoglobin 11–12.9 g/dL for men and 11–11.9 g/dL for women
Spontaneous bleeding requiring hospitalization or transfusion in the past 6 mo or at any time, if recurrent	Spontaneous bleeding requiring hospitalization or transfusion within the past 12 mo not meeting the major criterion
Moderate or severe baseline thrombocytopenia[b] (platelet count <100 × 10^9/L)	
Chronic bleeding diathesis	
Liver cirrhosis with portal hypertension	
	Long-term use of oral NSAIDs or steroids
Active malignancy[c] (excluding nonmelanoma skin cancer) within the past 12 mo	
Previous spontaneous ICH (at any time) Previous traumatic ICH within the past 12 mo Presence of a bAVM Moderate or severe ischemic stroke[d] within the past 6 mo	Any ischemic stroke at any time not meeting the major criterion
Nondeferrable major surgery on DAPT	
Recent major surgery or major trauma within 30 d before PCI	

Abbreviations: bAVM, brain arteriovenous malformation; CKD, chronic kidney disease; DAPT, dual antiplatelet therapy; eGFR, estimated glomerular filtration rate; HBR, high bleeding risk; ICH, intracranial hemorrhage; NSAID, nonsteroidal anti-inflammatory drug; PCI, percutaneous coronary intervention.

[a] This excludes vascular protection doses.
[b] Baseline thrombocytopenia is defined as thrombocytopenia before PCI.
[c] Active malignancy is defined as diagnosis within 12 mo and/or ongoing requirement for treatment (including surgery, chemotherapy, or radiotherapy).
[d] National Institutes of Health Stroke Scale score $\geq$5.
Adapted from Urban P, Mehran R, Colleran R, et al. Defining High Bleeding Risk in Patients Undergoing Percutaneous Coronary Intervention. *Circulation.* 2019;140(3):240-261; with permission.

THE LEADERS-FREE TRIALS

DES with durable polymers are associated with persistent fibrin deposition, greater inflammation, and poorer endothelialization, resulting in delayed arterial healing compared with BMS.[3] Both durable and biodegradable polymers have been associated with local arterial hypersensitivity reactions that may contribute to late thrombosis.[15,16] Therefore, a polymer-free stent that can successfully deliver an antiproliferative agent (a DCS) to minimize late loss may confer the efficacy of a DES without requiring long-term DAPT to mitigate the prolonged hazard of thrombotic risk associated with a drug-carrying polymer. The BioFreedom stent is a

PF-DCS that utilizes a modified BioFlex II metal platform and urolimus (biolimus A9, BA9). The stent is made of 316L stainless steel with a strut thickness of 112 μm; the abluminal side is modified to create a microstructured surface that enables BA9 to adhere to the stent without the use of a polymer (**Fig. 1**). Approximately 90% of the drug is released from the stent within 48 hours of implantation, with the remaining drug released within 28 days.[17,18] BA9 is a sirolimus analog that is a highly lipophilic, allowing for sustained retention within the intimal wall after its rapid release from the metal scaffold. The tissue concentration of BA9 in porcine arteries at 28 days after implantation of BioFreedom PF-DCS is comparable with that of durable polymer

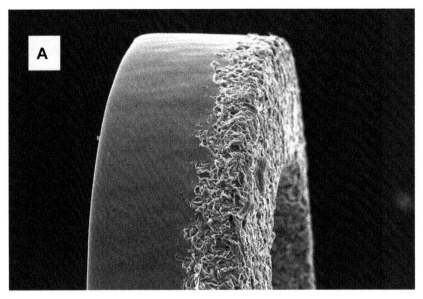

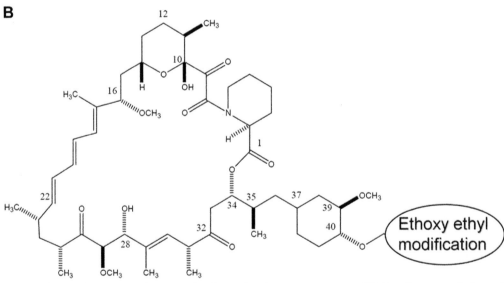

Fig. 1. The design of the BioFreedom stent. (*A*) Shows the electron microscopy of BioFreedom stent platform with a textured abluminal surface. (*B*) Shows molecular structure of BA9. (*From* Tada N, Virmani R, Grant G, et al. Polymer-free biolimus a9-coated stent demonstrates more sustained intimal inhibition, improved healing, and reduced inflammation compared with a polymer-coated sirolimus-eluting cypher stent in a porcine model. Circ Cardiovasc Interv 2010;3(2):174-83; with permission.)

DES.[18] In an early clinical study, the BioFreedom PF-DCS with a drug content of 15.6 μg/mm of stent length was associated with a late loss of only 0.17 mm at 1 year follow-up, which was noninferior to the comparator Taxus paclitaxel-eluting stent.[18]

LEADERS-FREE

The LEADERS-FREE trial was a randomized, double-blind, multicenter study designed to evaluate the clinical efficacy and safety of the

BioFreedom PF-DCS compared with a BMS (Gazelle, Biosensors International) in HBR patients with a 1-month course of DAPT in both groups.[12] The primary safety endpoint was a composite of cardiac death, MI or stent thrombosis, measured at 1-year follow-up. MI was defined according to the third universal definition.[19] The primary efficacy endpoint was clinically driven target lesion revascularization (TLR) at 1-year follow-up. HBR was based on the presence of one or more of the following criteria:

advanced age ($\geq$75 years), concurrent oral anti-coagulation, anemia (Hgb <11 g/L or transfusion within the prior month), thrombocytopenia (platelet count <100,000/mm^3), hospital admission for bleeding within the past year, stroke within the past year, previous intracranial hemorrhage, severe liver disease, renal dysfunction (creatine clearance <40 mL/min), cancer in the prior 3 years, planned major surgery in the next year, planned corticosteroid or nonsteroidal anti-inflammatory drug therapy for more than 30 days post-PCI, or expected nonadherence to more than 30 days of DAPT.

A total of 2466 patients were enrolled. Patients had a mean of 1.7 HBR inclusion criteria, the most frequent being age $\geq$75 years (64.3%), need for concurrent oral anticoagulation (36.1%), renal dysfunction (18.5%), planned major surgery within 12 months (16.4%), and anemia (15.6%). Nearly one-quarter of the enrolled patients presented with non-ST segment elevation MI, 15% with unstable angina, and 4.5% with ST segment elevation MI. Diabetes was present in approximately 33% of patients. More than 90% of the patients discontinued DAPT at 1-month after randomization, as mandated by the study protocol.

At 390-day follow-up, the BioFreedom PF-DCS was superior to BMS for the primary safety endpoint of cardiac death, MI, or stent thrombosis (9.4% versus 12.9%; HR = 0.71; 95% CI, 0.56–0.91; P = .005), driven by a lower rate of MI in the BioFreedom PF-DCS group (6.1% versus 8.9%; HR = 0.68; 95% CI, 0.50–0.91; P = .01). Both spontaneous MI (type I) and MI related to in-stent-restenosis (type 4c) were reduced with BioFreedom PF-DCS. The rates of definite or probable stent thrombosis were not different between groups (2.0% versus 2.2%; HR = 0.91; 95% CI, 0.53–1.59; P = .75). Subgroup analysis suggested a particular benefit with the BioFreedom DCS in patients without acute coronary syndrome (interaction P = .02), without anemia (interaction P = .03), and without renal dysfunction (interaction P = .02).

BioFreedom DCS was also associated with a significantly lower rate of the primary efficacy endpoint of clinically driven TLR at 1-year follow-up compared with the BMS control (5.1% versus 9.8%; HR = 0.50; 95% CI, 0.37–0.69; P<.001), consistent with the low rate of late loss observed in the BioFreedom First-in-Man (FIM) trial.[18] Urgent TLR, any TLR, and target vessel revascularization (TVR) were also reduced with BioFreedom DCS compared with BMS.

Bleeding was frequent and similar in both groups: the rate of BARC 3 or 5 bleeding at 1-

year follow-up was 7.2% with BioFreedom DCS and 7.3% with BMS (P = .96), consistent with the ARC definition of an HBR patient cohort ($\geq$4% BARC 3 or 5 bleeding at 1 year).[13]

The superiority of BioFreedom DCS over BMS was sustained at 2-year follow-up, with a significantly lower rate of the primary safety endpoint of cardiac death, MI, or stent thrombosis (12.6% versus 15.6%; HR = 0.80; 95% CI, 0.64–0.99; P = .039) and a significantly lower rate of clinically driven TLR (6.8% versus 12.0%; HR = 0.54; 95% CI, 0.41–0.72; P<.0001). Therefore, no "catch-up" effect was observed for TLR with the BioFreedom DCS beyond 1-year follow-up. The risk of all-cause death 1 year after a major bleed and 1 year after a coronary thrombotic event were similar and very high (27.1% and 26.3%, respectively), exemplifying the trade-off between a longer course of DAPT that might reduce thrombotic complications but likely increase the risk of major bleeding.[20]

LEADERS-FREE II

The LEADERS-FREE II study was designed to assess the reproducibility and generalizability of the benefits of the PF-DCS observed in the LEADERS-FREE in a predominantly North American cohort of HBR patients. LEADERS-FREE II was a prospective, multicenter, single-arm, open-label study. This design was chosen given the lack of equipoise to randomize against a BMS and the lack of any approved alternative device. Clinical inclusion and exclusion criteria, study definitions, and case report forms were identical to the LEADERS-FREE trial to enhance interpretability and comparison of the results between the studies. All patients were treated with low-dose aspirin and a P2Y$_{12}$ inhibitor (preferably clopidogrel) for 30 days. The primary safety endpoint was a combination of cardiac death and MI, and the primary efficacy endpoint was clinically driven TLR, both assessed at 1 year follow-up. The primary endpoints were compared with the BMS cohort of LEADERS-FREE using propensity-adjusted analyses for noninferiority and, if met, superiority.

A total of 1203 patients were enrolled, 761 in North America and 442 in Europe. Similar to LEADERS-FREE, patients displayed an average of 1.7 HBR inclusion criteria, and the 1-year rate of BARC 3 or 5 bleeding was 7.2%, identical to that observed in the BioFreedom PF-DCS arm of LEADERS-FREE. The rate of the primary safety endpoint of cardiac death or MI was noninferior and superior with BioFreedom PF-DCS compared with BMS (9.3% versus 12.4%; HR =

0.72; 95% CI, 0.55–0.94; $P<.001$ for noninferiority and $P = .015$ for superiority). Both components of the primary safety endpoint were lower with BioFreedom DCS (cardiac mortality, 3.5% versus 6.1%; HR = 0.70; 95% CI, 0.46–1.08; $P = .10$); MI 6.5% versus 8.8%, HR = 0.67 (95% CI, 0.49–0.92; $P = .01$). Definite or probable stent thrombosis was similar between the 2 arms (2.0% versus 2.2%). BioFreedom PF-DCS also met the noninferiority and superiority compared with BMS for primary efficacy endpoint of clinically driven TLR (7.2% versus 9.2%; HR = 0.72; 95% CI, 0.52–0.98; $P<.001$ for noninferiority, and $P = .0338$ for superiority).

Therefore, the LEADERS-FREE II study reproduced the results of the PF-DCS arm of the LEADERS-FREE trial in an independent, predominantly North American cohort of patients with HBR, supporting the contention that in HBR patients undergoing PCI, the use of BioFreedom PF-DCS followed by 30-day DAPT significantly reduces the composite of cardiac death and MI as well as clinically driven TLR at 1 year compared with BMS.

THE ONYX ONE TRIALS

Although the durable polymers of first-generation DES were associated with persistent inflammation, delayed endothelialization and late thrombotic events, post-hoc analyses of second generation DES, including the Resolute zotarolimus-eluting stent, suggest that early DAPT discontinuation between 1 and 12 months post-PCI may be safe.[21] The Resolute Onyx DES is an iteration of the Resolute DES family. A single, continuous strand of cobalt alloy wire material with a composite core of platinum and iridium with a swaged shape is formed into a sinusoidal design, helically wrapped around a mandril, and laser fused at specific crowns to form the final stent scaffold.[22,23] The strut thickness is 81 μm for the 2.0 to 4.0 mm diameter sizes. The Onyx DES features thinner struts than the predicate Resolute Integrity but with a larger strut width-to-thickness ratio to maintain radial strength and, like the previous Resolute stents, it elutes the mammalian target of rapamycin inhibitor zotarolimus from a durable BioLinx polymer. Almost 80% of the drug is released by 30 days, with the remainder eluted by 180 days.[24] In a small study of 15 patients undergoing Onyx DES implantation with 30-day follow-up optical coherence tomography, 92.3% of the total luminal surface was fully covered, suggesting rapid healing.[25]

ONYX ONE Trial

The ONYX ONE trial was a prospective, randomized, single-blinded trial designed to compare the safety and effectiveness of the durable polymer Onyx DES with the BioFreedom PF-DCS in HBR patients treated with 1-month of DAPT post-PCI.[14] The primary endpoint was a composite of cardiac death, MI, or definite/probable stent thrombosis assessed at 1-year follow-up. MI was defined according to the third universal definition.[19] The study was powered to determine noninferiority for the Onyx stent, assuming an expected rate of 9.4% for the BioFreedom PF-DCS and a noninferiority margin of 4.1%. The powered secondary endpoint was target lesion failure, a composite of cardiac death, target vessel MI, or clinically indicated TVR. This endpoint was powered for noninferiority, assuming an expected rate of 11% with BioFreedom PF-DCS and a noninferiority margin of 4.4%. Both endpoints were analyzed according to the intention-to-treat principle. To be enrolled, patients had to meet at least 1 specific criterion for HBR, similar to those of the LEADERS-FREE trial (Box 1).

A total of 3239 patients were enrolled at 83 sites outside the United States. Clinical characteristics reflected a group at significant ischemic risk: nearly 40% of the patients had diabetes, and the clinical presentation was non-ST segment elevation MI in 27% and ST segment elevation MI in 5.7%. The mean number of HBR criteria per patient was 1.6. The most frequent qualifying criteria were age ≥75 years (61.7% of patients), planned oral anticoagulation after PCI (38.5%), anemia (15.6%), and renal dysfunction (14.9%). Most lesions were complex (AHA/ACC B2/C class in 79.8%), and the average total stented length per patient was approximately 38 mm. Only 2 patients assigned to the Onyx DES crossed over to receive the BioFreedom PF-DCS, whereas 40 patients assigned to BioFreedom PF-DCS crossed over and received Onyx DES. Acute luminal gain and postprocedural percent diameter stenosis were superior with Onyx DES (1.72 ± 0.49 versus 1.67 ± 0.48, $P = .004$; 9.9 ± 8.7 versus 11.2 ± 9.4, $P<.001$), resulting in improved device success (achievement of <30% residual stenosis and Thrombolysis In Myocardial Infarction grade 3 flow using only the assigned device, 92.8% versus 89.7%, $P = .007$). The overwhelming majority of patients in both arms discontinued DAPT at 30 days and transitioned to single antiplatelet therapy (SAPT), consistent with the study protocol (at 2-month follow-up,

Box 1
High bleeding risk criteria required for inclusion in the ONYX ONE randomized clinical trial

- Age ≥75 years
- Adjunctive oral anticoagulation treatment planned to continue after PCI
- Baseline hemoglobin less than 11 g/dL, or anemia requiring transfusion during the 4 weeks before randomization
- Prior intracerebral bleed
- Any stroke within the last 12 months
- Hospital admission for bleeding during the previous 12 months
- Nonskin cancer diagnosed or treated with the past 3 years
- Planned daily nonsteroidal anti-inflammatory drug (other than aspirin) or steroids for ≥30 days after PCI
- Planned surgery that would require DAPT interruption within the next 12 months
- Renal dysfunction, defined as creatinine clearance <40 mL/min
- Thrombocytopenia, defined as platelet count less than 100,000/mm^3
- Severe liver disease
- Expected noncompliance to prolonged DAPT for other medical reasons.

Patients were required to fulfill one or more of these criteria.*Abbreviations:* DAPT, dual antiplatelet therapy; PCI, percutaneous coronary intervention.

92% of patients were on SAPT, 56% of whom were taking aspirin and 44% of were taking clopidogrel).

At 1-year follow-up, the rate of the primary endpoint of cardiac death, MI, or definite/probable stent thrombosis was 17.1% with Onyx DES and 16.9% with the BioFreedom PF-DCS, meeting the criteria for noninferiority (risk difference, 0.2%; upper boundary of the 1-sided 95% CI, 3.0; $P = .01$ for noninferiority). Onyx DES was also noninferior to the BioFreedom DCS for the powered, secondary effectiveness endpoint of TVF (17.6% versus 17.4%, risk difference, 0.2%; upper boundary of the 1-sided 95% CI, 3.0; $P = .007$ for noninferiority). Spontaneous MI occurred less frequently with the Onyx DES compared with BioFreedom DES (4.6% versus 7.1%, $P = .02$), although this observation must be interpreted cautiously. BARC type 3 to 5 bleeding occurred in 4.65% of patients by 1-

year follow-up, consistent with an HBR cohort as defined by the Academic Research Consortium.[13]

In summary, ONYX ONE demonstrated that among patients at HBR undergoing PCI who are treated with 1 month of DAPT, the Onyx DES had improved angiographic outcomes and device success compared with BioFreedom PF-DCS and was noninferior with respect to safety and effectiveness at 1-year follow-up.

ONYX ONE Clear

The ONYX ONE Clear (A Single Arm Study With Resolute Onyx in ONE-Month DAPT for High-Bleeding Risk Patients Who Are Considered One-Month Clear) study is a single-arm, open-label prospective study enrolling in the United States that is, evaluating the safety and effectiveness of the Onyx DES in HBR patients treated with 1-month of DAPT (clinicaltrials.gov identifier, NCT03647475). To be eligible, patients must be at HBR as defined by inclusion criteria similar to that of ONYX ONE and LEADERS-FREE. Approximately 750 patients will be enrolled. Patients will transition from DAPT to SAPT at 30 days if they have been compliant with DAPT and have not experienced a MACE or bleed ("clear"). The primary endpoint is a composite of cardiac death or MI between 1-month and 1-year in the clear population compared with a performance criterion. The results of this study will provide important data for 1-month DAPT after Onyx DES in HBR patients within the United States, and if consistent with the findings of ONYX ONE, provide greater support for abbreviated DAPT after PCI with Onyx DES in patients who are at particularly HBR.

Ongoing Studies of Abbreviated Dual Antiplatelet Therapy After Drug-Eluting Stents

Several other studies testing the safety and effectiveness of short-term DAPT after DES in HBR patients are planned or ongoing. The XIENCE 28 Global Study is a prospective, single-arm, nonrandomized study designed to evaluate the safety of the Xience everolimus-eluting stent (EES) (Abbott Vascular, Santa Clara, CA) in HBR patients treated with DAPT for 1-month; patients who are free from cardiac events and compliant with DAPT at 28 days will discontinue the P2Y$_{12}$ inhibitor and continue on maintenance dose aspirin (clinicaltrials.gov identifier, NCT03355742). Approximately 960 patients will be enrolled, and the primary endpoint is net adverse clinical events, consisting of the composite rate of all-cause death and MI, stent thrombosis, stroke or BARC type 2 to 5 bleeding. The EVOLVE (A Prospective Randomized Multicenter Single-Blind Noninferiority Trial to Assess the Safety and Performance of the Evolution Everolimus-Eluting Monorail Coronary Stent System for the Treatment of a De Novo Atherosclerotic Lesion) Short DAPT study (clinicaltrials.gov identifier, NCT02605447) will prospectively evaluate the safety of 3 months of DAPT in approximately 2000 HBR patients treated with the Synergy EES (Boston Scientific Corporation, Marlborough, MA). Patients free of events (stroke, MI, revascularization, or stent thrombosis) who discontinued $P2Y_{12}$ inhibitor at 3 months, but continued aspirin, will be assessed for 2 powered coprimary endpoints: (1) death or MI compared with a propensity-adjusted historical control, and (2) study stent-related definite or probable stent thrombosis compared with a performance goal.

Limitations of the Current Dataset

Although together the LEADERS-FREE and ONYX ONE provide the basis for abbreviated DAPT after PCI with PF-DCS or the Onyx zotarolimus-eluting stent, several limitations should be noted. Most importantly, the trials did not compare outcomes between a longer duration and an abbreviated duration of DAPT. The absolute rate of events between 1 and 12 months (ie, when patients were treated with SAPT) in both arms of ONYX ONE seem acceptable but may have been lower with the more prolonged duration of DAPT recommended by Society Guidelines.[7] Although the net clinical benefit of such an approach is an open question, the enrolled patients were generally not candidates for a longer regimen and are not reflected in contemporary stent trials on which the guidelines are in large part based. The findings of LEADERS-FREE and ONYX ONE should not be applied to patients who are not at HBR and who are good candidates for DAPT, as the ischemic benefit of prolonged DAPT, including reducing nonstent-related MACE,[4] may outweigh any small incremental risk of bleeding, particularly in those patients at high risk for ischemic events.[5,26,27]

SUMMARY

A cohort of patients can be identified as HBR based on a set of criteria that predict a major bleeding rate of $\geq$4% or a risk of intracranial hemorrhage of $\geq$1% per year. Such patients

have not been well represented in contemporary stent trials, which require subjects to be treated with a prolonged duration of DAPT. In the current era, approximately 20% of patients undergoing PCI receive a BMS, primarily due to bleeding risk or the need for surgery. The LEADERS-FREE trial demonstrated that a PF-DCS was safer and more effective than a BMS in patients at HBR undergoing PCI and treated with an abbreviated (1-month) duration of DAPT. The prospective, single-arm LEADERS-FREE II study provided supportive data for the PF-DCS in an independent, predominantly North American population. The ONYX ONE trial, building on the findings of LEADERS-FREE, demonstrated that the safety and effectiveness of the Onyx zotarolimus-eluting stent were noninferior to the PF-DCS in HBR patients treated with 1-month of DAPT, and the prospective, single-arm, ONYX ONE CLEAR study will further evaluate the Onyx stent with 1 month DAPT in an HBR population within the United States. Studies of abbreviated DAPT in HBR patients undergoing PCI with other newer-generation DES are ongoing. Risk stratification using the ARC HBR criteria and appropriate selection of a polymer-free drug-coated or durable polymer zotarolimus-eluting stent can optimize clinical outcomes in patients undergoing PCI who require an abbreviated DAPT regimen.

REFERENCES

1. Price MJ. The optimal duration of dual antiplatelet therapy after drug-eluting stent implantation: chasing a mirage. J Am Coll Cardiol 2015;65(13):1311–3.
2. Leon MB, Baim DS, Popma JJ, et al. A clinical trial comparing three antithrombotic-drug regimens after coronary-artery stenting. Stent Anticoagulation Restenosis Study Investigators. N Engl J Med 1998;339(23):1665–71.
3. Joner M, Finn AV, Farb A, et al. Pathology of drug-eluting stents in humans: delayed healing and late thrombotic risk. J Am Coll Cardiol 2006;48(1):193–202.
4. Mauri L, Kereiakes DJ, Yeh RW, et al. Twelve or 30 months of dual antiplatelet therapy after drug-eluting stents. N Engl J Med 2014;383:35–48..
5. Yeh RW, Kereiakes DJ, Steg PG, et al. Benefits and risks of extended duration dual antiplatelet therapy after PCI in patients with and without acute myocardial infarction. J Am Coll Cardiol 2015;65(20):2211–21.
6. Bonaca MP, Bhatt DL, Cohen M, et al. Long-term use of ticagrelor in patients with prior myocardial infarction. N Engl J Med 2015;372(19):1791–800.

7. Levine GN, Bates ER, Bittl JA, et al. 2016 ACC/AHA guideline focused update on duration of dual anti-platelet therapy in patients with coronary artery disease: a report of the American College of Cardiology/American Heart Association Task Force on Clinical Practice Guidelines: an update of the 2011 ACCF/AHA/SCAI guideline for percutaneous coronary intervention, 2011 ACCF/AHA guideline for coronary artery bypass graft surgery, 2012 ACC/AHA/ACP/AATS/PCNA/SCAI/STS guideline for the diagnosis and management of patients with stable ischemic heart disease, 2013 ACCF/AHA guideline for the management of ST-elevation myocardial infarction, 2014 AHA/ACC guideline for the management of patients with non-ST-elevation acute coronary syndromes, and 2014 ACC/AHA guideline on perioperative cardiovascular evaluation and management of patients undergoing noncardiac surgery. Circulation 2016; 134(10):e123–55.

8. Jensen CJ, Naber CK, Urban P, et al. 2-year outcomes of high bleeding risk patients with acute coronary syndrome after biolimus-A9 polymer-free drug-coated stents: a leaders free sub-study. EuroIntervention 2018. https://doi.org/10.4244/EIJ-D-17-00720.

9. Rymer JA, Harrison RW, Dai D, et al. Trends in bare-metal stent use in the United States in patients aged ≥65 years (from the CathPCI REGISTRY). Am J Cardiol 2016;118(7):959–66.

10. Shafiq A, Gosch K, Amin AP, et al. Predictors and variability of drug-eluting vs bare-metal stent selection in contemporary percutaneous coronary intervention: insights from the PRISM study. Clin Cardiol 2017;40(8):521–7.

11. Vora AN, Wang TY, Li S, et al. Selection of stent type in patients with atrial fibrillation presenting with acute myocardial infarction: an analysis from the ACTION (acute coronary treatment and intervention outcomes network) registry-get with the guidelines. J Am Heart Assoc 2017;6(8):e005280.

12. Urban P, Meredith IT, Abizaid A, et al. Polymer-free drug-coated coronary stents in patients at high bleeding risk. N Engl J Med 2015;373(21):2038–47.

13. Urban P, Mehran R, Colleran R, et al. Defining high bleeding risk in patients undergoing percutaneous coronary intervention. Circulation 2019;140(3):240–61.

14. Windecker S, Latib A, Kedhi E, et al. Polymer-based or polymer-free stents in patients at high bleeding risk. N Engl J Med 2020;382(13):1208–18.

15. Virmani R, Guagliumi G, Farb A, et al. Localized hypersensitivity and late coronary thrombosis secondary to a sirolimus-eluting stent: should we be cautious? Circulation 2004;109(6):701–5.

16. van der Giessen WJ, Lincoff AM, Schwartz RS, et al. Marked inflammatory sequelae to implantation of biodegradable and nonbiodegradable polymers in porcine coronary arteries. Circulation 1996; 94(7):1690–7.

17. Tada N, Virmani R, Grant G, et al. Polymer-free biolimus a9-coated stent demonstrates more sustained intimal inhibition, improved healing, and reduced inflammation compared with a polymer-coated sirolimus-eluting cypher stent in a porcine model. Circ Cardiovasc Interv 2010;3(2):174–83.

18. Costa RA, Abizaid A, Mehran R, et al. Polymer-free biolimus A9-coated stents in the treatment of De Novo coronary lesions: 4- and 12-month angiographic follow-up and final 5-year clinical outcomes of the prospective, multicenter BioFreedom FIM clinical trial. JACC Cardiovasc Interv 2016;9(1):51–64.

19. Thygesen K, Alpert JS, Jaffe AS, et al. Third universal definition of myocardial infarction. Circulation 2012;126(16):2020–35.

20. Garot P, Morice MC, Tresukosol D, et al. 2-year outcomes of high bleeding risk patients after polymer-free drug-coated stents. J Am Coll Cardiol 2017; 69(2):162–71.

21. Silber S, Kirtane AJ, Belardi JA, et al. Lack of association between dual antiplatelet therapy use and stent thrombosis between 1 and 12 months following resolute zotarolimus-eluting stent implantation. Eur Heart J 2014;35(29):1949–56.

22. Price MJ, Saito S, Shlofmitz RA, et al. First report of the resolute Onyx 2.0-mm zotarolimus-eluting stent for the treatment of coronary lesions with very small reference vessel diameter. JACC Cardiovasc Interv 2017;10(14):1381–8.

23. Price MJ, Shlofmitz RA, Spriggs DJ, et al. Safety and efficacy of the next generation resolute Onyx zotarolimus-eluting stent: primary outcome of the RESOLUTE ONYX core trial. Catheter Cardiovasc Interv 2018;92(2):253–9.

24. Kedhi E, Latib A, Abizaid A, et al. Rationale and design of the Onyx ONE global randomized trial: a randomized controlled trial of high-bleeding risk patients after stent placement with 1month of dual antiplatelet therapy. Am Heart J 2019;214:134–41.

25. Roleder T, Kedhi E, Berta B, et al. Short-term stent coverage of second-generation zotarolimus-eluting durable polymer stents: Onyx one-month optical coherence tomography study. Postepy Kardiol Interwencyjnej 2019;15(2):143–50.

26. Yeh RW, Secemsky EA, Kereiakes DJ, et al. Development and validation of a prediction rule for benefit and harm of dual antiplatelet therapy beyond 1 year after percutaneous coronary intervention. JAMA 2016;315(16):1735–49.

27. Costa F, van Klaveren D, James S, et al. Derivation and validation of the predicting bleeding complications in patients undergoing stent implantation and subsequent dual antiplatelet therapy (PRECISE-DAPT) score: a pooled analysis of individual-patient datasets from clinical trials. Lancet 2017;389(10073):1025–34.

Transcatheter Treatment of Functional Mitral Regurgitation in Patients with Heart Failure: The COAPT Trial

Nishtha Sodhi, MD[a],*, David Scott Lim, MD[a,b]

KEYWORDS

- Functional mitral regurgitation • COAPT • MitraClip • Transcatheter mitral valve repair
- Congestive heart failure

KEY POINTS

- Functional mitral regurgitation (FMR) is strongly associated with recurrent heart failure (HF) hospitalizations, poor quality of life, and poor prognosis, and the 5-year mortality in patients with severe symptomatic FMR is nearly as high as 60%; current goals of therapy for these patients rest on guideline-directed medical therapy (GDMT) targeting the underlying left ventricular dysfunction.
- COAPT was a multicenter, randomized, parallel-controlled, open-label multicenter trial of transcatheter mitral valve leaflet repair (TMVr) with the MitraClip device in patients with HF and at least moderate-to-severe MR with at least New York Heart Association class II symptoms despite stable GDMT irrespective of surgical risk.
- The COAPT trial demonstrated that TMVr decreases the severity of FMR, lowers the rate of hospitalization for heart failure and the rate of mortality, and improves quality of life and functional capacity compared with GDMT alone.
- The benefits of TMVr were demonstrated across ischemic versus nonischemic causes, HF with reduced (left ventricular ejection fraction [LVEF]≤40%) and preserved EF (LVEF≥40% and <50%), and across the spectrum of surgical risk.
- Creation of stenosis with mean mitral gradient up to 7 mm Hg after MitraClip did not diminish the improvement in outcomes, suggesting that the benefits of MR reduction outweigh the effects of mild-to-moderate mitral stenosis.

INTRODUCTION

Mitral regurgitation (MR) is the most common valvular heart disease with a prevalence of nearly 10% in individuals older than 75 years.[1] MR is broadly differentiated by primary valvular versus secondary functional causes. Primary MR describes degenerative abnormalities of the valvular apparatus itself, including the leaflets, chordae tendineae, papillary muscles, or mitral annulus. Functional MR (FMR) describes regurgitation caused by the secondary effects of left ventricular (LV) dysfunction and dilation despite a normal mitral valve (MV) apparatus. In the cardiomyopathic heart, leaflet tethering and geometric dislocation of the papillary muscles and chordae tendineae result in impaired leaflet coaptation and late annular dilation.[1–4] A subset

[a] Division of Cardiovascular Medicine, Department of Medicine, Advanced Cardiac Valve Center, University of Virginia, 1215 Lee Street, Charlottesville, VA 22909, USA; [b] Division of Pediatric Cardiology, Department of Pediatrics, Advanced Cardiac Valve Center, University of Virginia, 1215 Lee Street, Charlottesville, VA 22909, USA
* Corresponding author.
E-mail address: NS9SA@hscmail.mcc.virginia.edu
Twitter: @NishthaSodhi (N.S.)

Intervent Cardiol Clin 9 (2020) 451–459
https://doi.org/10.1016/j.iccl.2020.07.001
2211-7458/20/© 2020 Elsevier Inc. All rights reserved.

of FMR, atrial FMR, describes secondary MR in the setting of atrial remodeling and annular dilation secondary to atrial fibrillation but is associated with preserved LV size and systolic function.

BACKGROUND

According to the latest American Heart Association (AHA) data, FMR is present in 16,250 per million people in the United States, with an incidence and prevalence predicted to increase with the increase in the aging population and incidence of heart failure (HF).[2,5]

FMR is strongly associated with increased all-cause mortality and HF hospitalizations along with decreased quality of life.[4,6] Among 404 consecutive patients with severe FMR treated with guideline directed medical therapy (GDMT), Agricola and colleagues found that 4-year cardiac mortality occurred in 43% and 45% with moderate and severe MR, respectively, compared with only 6% with mild MR (P<.003).[7] In a study from the Duke Cardiovascular Databank, 3+ to 4+ MR on left ventriculography was present in 30% of 2057 patients with HF with a left ventricular ejection fraction (LVEF) less than 40% and was an independent predictor of 5-year mortality (adjusted hazard ratio [HR]: 1.23; 95% confidence interval [CI], 1.13–1.34).[8] A Mayo Clinic study reported similar results with severe secondary MR as an independent predictor of death or HF hospitalization at median 2.5-year follow-up (adjusted HR: 1.5; 95% CI, 1.2–1.9), independent of LVEF.[9] However, until recently, it was unknown whether prognosis and severity of MR were mere associations or whether reducing the degree of MR severity could directly improve prognosis.

Goals of FMR therapy are to reduce HF hospitalizations, improve quality of life and symptoms, and potentially improve survival. As such, GDMT for HF with beta-blockade, angiotensin-converting enzyme inhibitors, and aldosterone antagonism, along with biventricular pacing, if applicable, have been the cornerstones in efforts to improve LV dysfunction and symptoms.

Although surgery is often curative for primary degenerative MR, surgery for FMR remains suboptimal. Surgical options for FMR include surgical MV repair and replacement, implantation of mechanical LV assist devices, and heart transplant.[4] Historically, surgical MV replacement with extensive excision of the leaflets and subvalvular apparatus was performed, but this resulted in annular-ventricular dyssynchrony and frequently resulted in decompensation.[4] If replacement is unavoidable, chordal-sparing MV replacement is now preferred, albeit compared with repair techniques, replacement is associated with higher perioperative mortality but lower recurrence in MR. Indeed, surgical repair with ring annuloplasty improves regurgitation in the short term, but recurrent MR is frequent.

Controversy exists regarding which surgical strategy is most appropriate for FMR. The Cardiothoracic Surgical Trials Network studied 251 patients with severe ischemic MR who were randomized to undergo either MV repair with an undersized rigid or semirigid complete annuloplasty ring or chordal-sparing MV replacement.[10] However, recurrence of at least moderate MR at 1 year was substantially greater with MV repair compared with replacement (33% vs 2%, P < .001).[10] In the 2-year follow-up analysis of this study, 59% of the patients in the repair group had recurrence of moderate-to-severe MR compared with 4% in the replacement group.[11] Given these data, many patients do not undergo surgical repair or replacement of isolated secondary MR. In fact, there is only a class IIb level of evidence B designation in the 2017 AHA/American College of Cardiology (AHA/ACC) Guidelines for isolated MV surgery.[12] Accordingly, there is a significant patient cohort that could benefit from alternative therapies, particularly transcatheter therapies designed to emulate surgical techniques. Thus emerged the MitraClip device (Abbott Vascular, Santa Clara, CA, USA) designed as the transcatheter rendition of the surgical Alfieri stitch to create a double orifice mitral valve.

MitraClip DEVICE AND PROCEDURE

The MitraClip device is composed of an implanted polyester-covered cobalt-chromium clip along with clip delivery system and steerable guide sheath (Fig. 1). The procedure is performed under general anesthesia and transesophageal echocardiographic guidance, with femoral venous access followed by transseptal puncture to introduce the steerable guide sheath into the left atrium through which the clip delivery system is advanced and introduced. The MitraClip is aligned coaxial to the mitral valve orifice and positioned over the regurgitant jet and then advanced into the LV. It is then retracted to grasp the free edges of the mitral leaflets, the frictional gripper elements are lowered to secure the leaflets, and the clip is closed and released. Before final deployment, leaflet insertion, tissue bridging, and hemodynamic assessments are performed to ensure that both leaflets are secured and that there is no

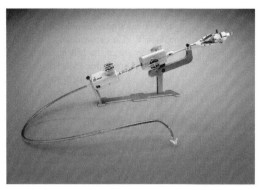

Fig. 1. The MitraClip device. (MitraClip is a trademark of Abbott or its related companies. Reproduced with permission of Abbott, © 2020. All rights reserved.)

inadvertent creation of mitral stenosis for the degree of MR reduction. Multiple clips may be implanted depending on the complexity of the mitral anatomy.

COAPT TRIAL RATIONALE

In the EVEREST II (Endovascular Valve Edge-to-Edge Repair Study) trial, 278 relatively low-risk patients with 3 to 4+ MR (73% primary MR) were randomized to MitraClip or surgical MV repair.[13] Compared with mitral surgery, the MitraClip was substantially safer but not as effective in reducing MR and LV remodeling.[13] Nonetheless, with follow-up to 4 years, New York Heart Association (NYHA) functional class and overall survival were similar in both groups.[14] This led the United States Food and Drug Administration (FDA) to approve the MitraClip in 2013 for primary MR patients deemed to be at prohibitive surgical risk by a multidisciplinary heart team. However, from the EVEREST II data, it was unclear whether solely reducing FMR with the MitraClip in the presence of underlying LV dysfunction would improve prognosis and quality of life. This question provided the justification for further study of the MitraClip's safety and efficacy in FMR and set the stage for the COAPT trial (The Cardiovascular Outcomes Assessment of the MitraClip Percutaneous Therapy for Heart Failure patients with Functional Mitral Regurgitation, ClinicalTrials.gov Identifier: NCT01626079).

COAPT STUDY DESIGN AND OBJECTIVES

COAPT was a randomized, parallel-controlled, open-label multicenter trial of transcatheter MV repair (TMVr) with the MitraClip device in patients with HF and at least 3+ or greater MR

with at least NYHA class II symptoms despite stable GDMT.[6,15] The study was funded by Abbott Vascular and designed in concert with the FDA and in accordance with the principles delineated by the Mitral Valve Academic Research Consortium. Both ischemic and nonischemic cardiomyopathies with LVEF of 20% to 50% with at least moderate-to-severe MR were evaluated by the heart team.[15]

Because of the potential heterogeneity in assessing FMR due to a wide variety of regurgitant orifice shapes, dynamic changes throughout the cardiac cycle, and suboptimal views and inconsistent reproducibility, the COAPT trial implemented a tiered echocardiographic assessment algorithm as shown in **Fig. 2**.[16] Principal echocardiographic exclusion criterion included less than 3+ MR severity, primary or mixed MR cause, left ventricular end-systolic diameter (LVESD) greater than 70 mm, and LVEF less than 20% or greater than 50%.[16]

Patients were randomized in a 1:1 fashion to TMVr with MitraClip device and GDMT versus GDMT alone. Key exclusion criteria were EF less than 20%, LVESD greater than or equal to 70 mm, ACC/AHA stage D HF, hemodynamic instability requiring inotropic support or mechanical heart assistance, evidence of right-sided congestive HF with echocardiographic evidence of moderate or severe right ventricular dysfunction, and estimated pulmonary artery systolic pressure greater than 70 mm Hg, unless active vasodilator therapy was able to reduce the pulmonary vascular resistance to less than 4.5 Wood units with v wave less than twice the mean of the pulmonary capillary wedge pressure.[15–17] Thus, stable but declining patients were considered but not those in cardiogenic shock who otherwise had no surgical options.

PRIMARY EFFECTIVENESS AND SAFETY ENDPOINTS

The primary powered effectiveness endpoint was hospitalizations for HF within 24 months of follow-up, including recurrent events in patients with more than one event.[15] This analysis was performed in the intention-to-treat population. The primary powered safety end point was freedom from device-related complications at 12 months compared with a performance goal. A device-related complication was defined as any occurrence of single-leaflet device attachment, device embolization, endocarditis requiring surgery, echocardiographic core laboratory confirmed mitral stenosis that required surgery, LV assist device implantation, heart

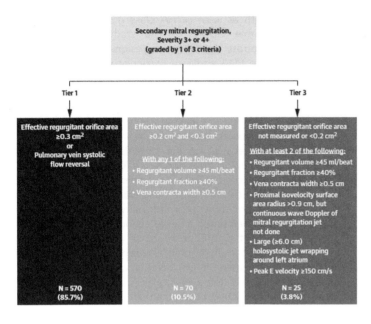

Fig. 2. This multiparametric screening algorithm was used by the COAPT (Cardiovascular Outcomes Assessment of the MitraClip Percutaneous Therapy for Heart Failure Patients with Functional Mitral Regurgitation) trial echocardiography core laboratory to determine if baseline mitral regurgitation severity was 3+ or higher for qualification purposes. The 3 tiers of evaluation were applied in a hierarchical manner (from tier 1–3); patients qualified for COAPT by meeting criteria of at least 1 of them. Mitral regurgitation severity was subsequently graded as 3+ versus 4+ based on the integrative evaluation of multiple parameters recommended by the American Society of Echocardiography guidelines. (*From* Asch FM, Grayburn PA, Siegel RJ, et al. Citation: Echocardiographic Outcomes After Transcatheter Leaflet Approximation in Patients With Secondary Mitral Regurgitation: The COAPT Trial. J Am Coll Cardiol 2019;74:2969-3679; with permission.)

transplant, or any other device-related event that led to nonelective cardiovascular surgery.[15] This analysis was performed in the safety analysis population, which was defined as all randomized device group patients in whom the MitraClip was attempted.[6,15]

RESULTS

Between 2012 and 2017, the echocardiographic core laboratory reviewed 1576 patients from 78 centers in the United States and Canada. A total 614 patients were eventually randomized, in addition to 51 roll-ins[6,15,16]; 302 patients were randomly assigned to the device group and 312 to the control group. Among the 665 enrolled patients, 85.7% met the $\geq$3+ MR severity criteria based on the first tier of the multiparameter algorithm, whereas the remainder qualified based on tiers 2 or 3.[6,15,16]

The mean ($\pm$SD) age was 72.2 $\pm$ 11.2 years and only 36.0% were women.[15] Ischemic cardiomyopathy was the cause in 60.7% of the patients and nonischemic in 39.3%. The mean LVEF was 31.3 $\pm$ 9.3%, and the MR grade was 3+ in 52.2% of the patients and 4+ in 47.8%. The mean Society of Thoracic Surgeons score for the risk of death within 30 days after mitral valve replacement was 8.2 $\pm$ 5.9%. Device implantation was attempted in 293 of the 302 patients (97.0%) in the device group, with 1 or more clips implanted in 287 patients (98.0% of the 293 patients in whom implantation was attempted).[15]

As seen in Fig. 3, the annualized rate of all hospitalizations for HF was 35.8% per patient-year in the TMVr group as compared with 67.9% per patient-year in the control group (HR, 0.53; 95% CI, 0.40–0.70; P<.001).[15] Impressively, the number needed to treat (NNT) to prevent 1 hospitalization for HF within 24 months was 3.1 (95% CI, 1.9–7.9).[15] Of note, the lower rate of hospitalization for HF with TMVr emerged within 30 days after treatment, whereas the lower mortality predominantly emerged more than 1 year after treatment. These findings are consistent with acute improvements in symptoms and quality of life and more durable improvements in LV remodeling and volume secondary to decreased severity of LV volume overload.

All-cause mortality within 24 months was significantly lower in the TMVr MitraClip-treated group than with medical therapy alone (29.1% vs 46.1%; HR, 0.62; 95% CI, 0.46–0.82; P<.001).[15] Remarkably, the NNT to save one life within 24 months was 5.9 (95% CI, 3.9–11.7).[15] Finally, quality of life, functional capacity, MR, and LV remodeling all improved in the TMVr arm, whereas there was no improvement in the GDMT arm.[15]

DISCUSSION

FMR is well correlated with recurrent HF hospitalizations, poor quality of life, and poor prognosis. The 5-year mortality in patients with severe symptomatic FMR is nearly as high as 60%.[8] Aside from the morbidity and mortality,

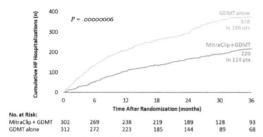

Fig. 3. Results from COAPT Trial with endpoints of heart failure hospitalization. (COAPT and MitraClip are trademarks of Abbott or its related companies. Reproduced with permission of Abbott, © 2020. All rights reserved.)

the associated economic and health-care resource utilization burden is substantial.[6] As such, the goals of therapy for these patients had been previously resting on GDMT targeting the underlying LV dysfunction. However, until the COAPT trial, it was unclear whether an intervention that reduces FMR in patients with primary LV dysfunction will improve patient outcomes.

COAPT revealed that in patients with HF, treatment with the MitraClip device had high procedural success rates and low procedural complication rates. Those patients who had lower residual MR did better compared with patients who remained with greater than 2+ residual MR.[18] These patients had more significant reduction in LV volumes and dimensions and more significant reduction in mitral valve annular dimensions. Thus, improvement in FMR and subsequent LV remodeling translated into improvement in prognosis, quality of life, and functional capacity. Indeed, device therapy resulted in a significantly lower rate of hospitalization for HF, lower mortality, and better quality of life and functional capacity within 24 months of follow-up compared with medical therapy alone. Furthermore, these benefits prevailed across ischemic versus nonischemic causes, HF with reduced ejection fraction (HFrEF) (LVEF<40%) and HF with preserved ejection fraction (HFpEF) (LVEF>40%), and in those with severe (LVEF<30%) and moderate (LVEF>30%) LV dysfunction.[19,20] In addition, creation of stenosis with mean mitral gradient up to 7 mm Hg after MitraClip did not impair these outcomes, suggesting that the benefits of MR reduction outweigh the effects of mild-to-moderate mitral stenosis.[21] For the first time, tangible benefits to prevent HF hospitalization and improve mortality in patients with MR were observed compared with GDMT alone.

At 3-year follow-up, the Kaplan Meier curves for the primary endpoint of death and HF hospitalizations for the intention-to-treat groups continued to separate, reaching 88% for the GDMT group and 58.8% in the MitraClip group.[22] The NNT declined from 4.5 at 2 years to 3.4 at 3 years.[22] Crossover from GDMT to TMVr was allowed after the initial 24-month period. Although many patients in the GDMT arm died before 2 years, 38% patients initially in the GDMT arm underwent TMVr between 24 and 36 months and had similar benefits to the original TMVr arm, with fewer HF-related hospitalization and death or HF hospitalizations within 12 months, compared with patients who did not crossover.[22]

Patients with high pulmonary artery systolic pressures (PASP>50 mm Hg) had higher 2-year rates of death or HF hospitalization compared with those patients with PASP less than 50 mm Hg.[15,23] However, TMVr reduced PASP from baseline to 30 days to a greater degree than GDMT.[23] Furthermore, reduction in PASP at 30 days was independently associated with reduced risk of death or HF hospitalization between 30 days and 2 years.[23]

Right ventricular systolic pressures (>45 mm Hg), 2+ or greater TR, and LVESD greater than 5.5 cm were significant predictive of adverse outcomes of death or HF hospitalization in GDMT-treated patients.[16,23,24] Indeed, a COAPT risk score has been developed to predict future risk of death and HF hospitalization at 2 years and includes the aforementioned variables as well as chronic kidney disease stage III or greater and atrial fibrillation and flutter.[24] Patients with atrial fibrillation likely represented FMR secondary to a mixture of atrial and ventricular remodeling. Although these patients had overall worse prognosis, they still derived benefit from TMVr and even had reduced stroke risk.[25]

The potential implications of this treatment strategy could transform the disease management for this cohort of patients who otherwise have limited options. Patient selection is key, and not all patients with FMR will benefit as described in the next section.

COAPT TRIAL: CLINICAL CONTEXT

Amid the release of COAPT, another trial examining TMVr, MITRA-FR (Percutaneous Repair or Medical Treatment for Secondary Mitral Regurgitation) had contrary results.[26] This trial performed in France intended to treat patients with severe FMR in a 1:1 ratio to undergo

TMVr with MitraClip along with GDMT versus GDMT alone. The primary efficacy outcome was a composite of death from any cause or unplanned hospitalization for HF at 12 months. Severe MR was defined as effective regurgitant orifice area (EROA) of greater than 20 mm^2 or a regurgitant volume of greater than 30 mL per beat and LVEF between 15% and 40%.[26] At 12 months, the rate of the primary outcome was 54.6% (83 of 152 patients) in the TMVr group and 51.3% (78 of 152 patients) in the control group (odds ratio, 1.16; 95% CI, 0.73–1.84; $P = .53$).[26] The rate of death from any cause was 24.3% (37 of 152 patients) in the TMVr group and 22.4% (34 of 152 patients) in the control group (HR, 1.11; 95% CI, 0.69–1.77).[26] The rate of unplanned hospitalization for HF was 48.7% (74 of 152 patients) in the TMVr group and 47.4% (72 of 152 patients) in the control group (HR, 1.13; 95% CI, 0.81–1.56).[26] Given these data, the investigators concluded that 1-year rates of unplanned HF admission and rate of death were not improved with TMVr combined with GDMT versus GDMT alone.

With nearly opposing results from 2 published trials examining TMVr, many investigators sought to explain and account for the differences. Using the Gorlin hydraulic formula, Grayburn and colleagues demonstrated that in a patient with typical HF with LVEDV 220 to 250 mL and a regurgitant fraction of 50%, which is the definition of severe MR, the EROA ranged from 0.3 to 0.35 cm^2.[27] When compared with the average EROA and LVEDV in COAPT versus MITRA-FR, there is a significant difference shown in Fig. 4, which likely explains the opposing outcomes in part.[27] COAPT patients had an EROA approximately 30% higher and with LV volumes approximately 30% smaller, that is, disproportionately more severe FMR than expected for the degree of LV chamber dilation.[27] This is in contrast to the MITRA-FR patient who had FMR severity that was proportionate and correlative for the degree of LV chamber dilation, that is, proportionately severe FMR. Additional differences include less stringent GDMT, relative technical inexperience, worse procedural outcomes, and incomplete echocardiographic follow-up data in MITRA-FR. Thus, these trials taken together, suggest that those patients with disproportionately severe FMR, rather than patients with proportionately severe FMR, benefit more from TMVr with MitraClip, which potentially explains why COAPT showed benefit.[27]

COAPT TRIAL: CLINICAL IMPACT

COAPT and MITRA-FR have helped to improve our understanding of FMR and which of those patients will benefit from TMVr. Disproportionate FMR has emerged as a term to define patients with more severe MR for the degree of LV dilation, whereas proportionate FMR describes MR severity that correlates to the degree of LV dysfunction and dilation. The appropriate TMVr candidate is thus one with disproportionately severe MR with indexed LV end-diastolic volumes that are not markedly dilated (mean LVEDV 101 mL/m^2 in COAPT) as outlined in the trial inclusion and echocardiographic criteria (see Fig. 2).[27] Foremost in the care of all of these patients is optimal GDMT and care by a multidisciplinary heart team including HF specialists. For the appropriate candidate, the improvement in MR severity after TMVr was durable throughout the 24-month follow-up. Furthermore, TMVr achieved remarkably low NNT to reduce HF hospitalization and mortality at 24 months. These benefits prevailed across ischemic versus nonischemic causes, HFrEF and HFpEF, and in those with severe and moderate LV dysfunction.[19,20] In addition, creation of stenosis with mean mitral gradient up to 7 mm Hg after MitraClip did not impair these outcomes, suggesting that the benefits of MR reduction outweigh the effects of mild-to-moderate mitral stenosis. For the first time, tangible benefits to prevent HF hospitalization and improve mortality in patients with MR were observed compared with GDMT alone.

Given the economic and health care burden of increasing HF costs, Baron and colleagues analyzed the cost-effectiveness of device therapy and found that TMVr reduced follow-up costs by greater than $11,000/patient compared with GDMT alone.[28–35] Although there are higher upfront costs during the index hospitalization, over a lifetime horizon, TMVr was projected to increase quality-adjusted life expectancy (QALY) by 0.82 at an incremental cost of $45,548, yielding a lifetime incremental cost-effectiveness ratio of $55,600 QALY gained.[28] Based on currently accepted US health care economic thresholds, TMVr is thus consistent with intermediate-to-high economic value.

TMVr may signal a paradigm shift in the care of patients with FMR. COAPT showed for the first time that treating MR in patients with HF resulted in reduction in HF hospitalization and all-cause mortality.[17] Indeed, MitraClip has emerged as the control group in upcoming transcatheter mitral trials in FMR and may represent a new standard of care. The FDA approved

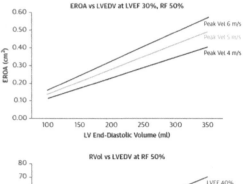

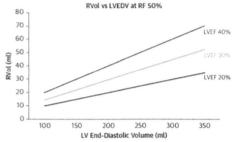

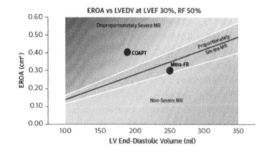

Fig. 4. Delineation of domains to identify patients with (1) nonsevere MR; (2) severe MR that is proportional to left ventricular end-diastolic volume (LVEDV); and (3) severe MR that is disproportionate to LVEDV. The diagram depicts the relation between effective regurgitant orifice area (EROA) and LVEDV, assuming an LVEF of 30% with a regurgitant fraction of 50%. (*Blue line*) The hypothetical relationship when the degree of severe MR is proportional to the LVEDV. (*Gray area*) A degree of uncertainty that is determined by the imprecision inherent in the measurement of EROA as well as the hemodynamic state of the patient. (*Pink area in the upper left*) Severe MR that is disproportionate to LV dilation. (*Green area in the lower right*) Nonsevere MR. (*Red dots*) The average patient enrolled in the MITRA-FR and COAPT trials, based on the information made public to date. (*From* Grayburn PA, Sannino A, Packer M. Proportionate and Disproportionate Functional Mitral Regurgitation: A New Conceptual Framework That Reconciles the Results of the MITRA-FR and COAPT Trials. JACC Cardiovasc Imaging. 2019 Feb;12(2):353-362; with permission.)

MitraClip based on the COAPT results in March of 2019 for treatment of moderate-to-severe and severe FMR despite GDMT.

SUMMARY

In COAPT, patients with HF and moderate-to-severe or severe FMR who remained symptomatic despite the use of maximal doses of GDMT benefited from MitraClip. The improvement in MR was durable through 24 months. Indeed, patients treated with MitraClip had a lower rate of hospitalization for HF, lower mortality, and better quality of life and functional capacity within 24 months of follow-up than medical therapy alone, and the prespecified goal for freedom from device-related complications was met. The COAPT trial has transformed the treatment toolbox for patients with FMR who otherwise have limited options.

DISCLOSURE

Dr N. Sodhi reports that she has nothing to disclose. Dr S. Lim reports that on his behalf his institution has received research funding from Abbott Vascular, Ancora Heart, Edwards Lifesciences, Medtronic. He also reports consulting income from Abbott Vascular (minimal) and Edwards Lifesciences (minimal).

REFERENCES

1. Nkomo VT, Gardin JM, Skelton TN, et al. Burden of valvular heart diseases: a population-based study. Lancet 2006;368:1005–11.
2. de Marchena E, Badiye A, Robalino G, et al. Respective prevalence of the different Carpentier classes of mitral regurgitation: a stepping stone for future therapeutic research and development. J Card Surg 2011;26:385–92.
3. Hung J, Papakostas L, Tahta SA, et al. Mechanism of recurrent ischemic mitral regurgitation after annuloplasty: continued LV remodeling as a moving target. Circulation 2004;110:II85–90.
4. Asgar AW, Mack MJ, Stone GW. Secondary mitral regurgitation in heart failure: pathophysiology, prognosis, and therapeutic considerations. J Am Coll Cardiol 2015;65(12):1231–48.
5. Benjamin EJ, Virani SS, Callaway CW, et al. Heart Disease and Stroke Statistics-2018 Update: A

Report From the American Heart Association. Circulation 2018;137:e67–492.

6. Mack MJ, Abraham WT, Lindenfeld J, et al. Cardiovascular Outcomes Assessment of the MitraClip in Patients with Heart Failure and Secondary Mitral Regurgitation: Design and rationale of the COAPT trial. Am Heart J 2018;205:1–11.

7. Agricola E, Ielasi A, Oppizzi M, et al. Long-term prognosis of medically treated patients with functional mitral regurgitation and left ventricular dysfunction. Eur J Heart Fail 2009;11:581–7.

8. Trichon BH, Felker GM, Shaw LK, et al. Relation of frequency and severity of mitral regurgitation to survival among patients with left ventricular systolic dysfunction and heart failure. Am J Cardiol 2003;91: 538–43.

9. Rossi A, Dini FL, Faggiano P, et al. Independent prognostic value of functional mitral regurgitation in patients with heart failure. A quantitative analysis of 1256 patients with ischaemic and nonischaemic dilated cardiomyopathy. Heart 2011;97:1675–80.

10. Acker MA, Parides MK, Perrault LP, et al. for the CTSN Investigators. Mitral-valve repair versus replacement for severe ischemic mitral regurgitation. N Engl J Med 2014;370:23–32.

11. Goldstein D, Moskowitz AJ, Gelijns AC, et al. Two-Year Outcomes of Surgical Treatment of Severe Ischemic Mitral Regurgitation. N Engl J Med 2016;374(4):344–53.

12. Nishimura RA, Otto CM, Bonow RO, et al. 2017 AHA/ACC Focused Update of the 2014 AHA/ACC Guideline for the Management of Patients With Valvular Heart Disease: A Report of the American College of Cardiology/American Heart Association Task Force on Clinical Practice Guidelines. J Am Coll Cardiol 2017;70(2):252–89.

13. Feldman T, Foster E, Glower DD, et al, for the EVEREST II Investigators. Percutaneous repair or surgery for mitral regurgitation. N Engl J Med 2011;364:1395–406.

14. Mauri L, Foster E, Glower DD, et al. 4-year results of a randomized controlled trial of percutaneous repair versus surgery for mitral regurgitation. J Am Coll Cardiol 2013;62:317–28.

15. Stone GW, Lindenfeld J, Abraham WT, et al. Transcatheter mitral-valve repair in patients with heart failure. N Engl J Med 2018;379(24):2307–18.

16. Asch FM, Grayburn PA, Siegel RJ, et al. Echocardiographic outcomes after transcatheter leaflet approximation in patients with secondary mitral regurgitation: the COAPT trial. J Am Coll Cardiol 2019;74(24):2969–79.

17. Goel K. Secondary MR: How has the COAPT Trial changed our approach?. Available at: https://www.acc.org/latest-in-cardiology/articles/2019/05/10/14/40/secondary-mr. Accessed March 31, 2020.

18. Kar S. Relationship between residual mitral regurgitation and clinical and functional outcomes in the COAPT trial. Presented at: EuroPCR 2019. Paris, France, May 21, 2019.

19. Lerakis, et al. Outcomes of transcatheter mitral valve repair in patients with secondary mitral regurgitation according to the severity of left ventricular dysfunction: the COAPT Trial. Poster presented at American College of Cardiology Conference. 2020.

20. Al-Azizi K, Grayburn PA, Szerlip M, et al. Outcomes of transcatheter mitral valve repair in ischemic versus non-ischemic cardiomyopathy: the COAPT Trial. J Am Coll Cardiol 2020;75(11 Supplement 1):1178.

21. Halaby R, Herrmann H, Lim S, et al. Lack of association of mitral valve gradient after MitraClip with outcomes in functional mitral regurgitation: results from COAPT Trial. J Am Coll Cardiol 2020;75(11 Supplement 1):1309.

22. Mack M, Abraham WT, Lindenfeld J, et al. Three-year outcomes from a randomized trial of transcatheter mitral valve leaflet approximation in patients with heart failure and secondary mitral regurgitation. Transcatheter Cardiovascular Therapeutics Conference 2019. San Francisco, California.

23. Ben-Yehuda, et al. Impact of Pulmonary Hypertension in Patients undergoing Transcatheter Mitral Valve Repair for Secondary Mitral Regurgitation: The COAPT Trial. Poster presented at American College of Cardiology Conference. 2020.

24. Shah, N, et al. Predictors of Death or HF Hospitalization in Patients with Functional Mitral Regurgitation. Poster presented at American College of Cardiology Conference. 2020.

25. Gertz Z, Herrmann H, Lim S, et al. Impact of a history of atrial fibrillation on the mechanism of mitral regurgitation, prognosis and treatment effects of the MitraClip: The COAPT Trial. J Am Coll Cardiol 2020;75(11 Supplement 1):1171.

26. Obadia JF, Messika-Zeitoun D, Leurent G, et al. Percutaneous Repair or Medical Treatment for Secondary Mitral Regurgitation. N Engl J Med 2018; 379(24):2297–306.

27. Grayburn PA, Sannino A, Packer M. Proportionate and Disproportionate Functional Mitral Regurgitation: A New Conceptual Framework That Reconciles the Results of the MITRA-FR and COAPT Trials. JACC Cardiovasc Imaging 2019;12(2): 353–62.

28. Baron SJ, Wang K, Arnold SV, et al. Cost-Effectiveness of Transcatheter Mitral Valve Repair Versus Medical Therapy in Patients With Heart Failure and Secondary Mitral Regurgitation: Results From the COAPT Trial. Circulation 2019;140(23): 1881–91.

29. Sannino A, Smith RL II, Schiattarella GG, et al. Survival and cardiovascular outcomes of patients with

secondary mitral regurgitation: a systematic review and metaanalysis. JAMA Cardiol 2017;2:1130–9.

30. Stone GW, Vahanian AS, Adams DH, et al. Clinical trial design principles and endpoint definitions for transcatheter mitral valve repair and replacement: Part 1: clinical trial design principles — a consensus document from the Mitral Valve Academic Research Consortium. J Am Coll Cardiol 2015;66:278–307.

31. Goel SS, Bajaj N, Aggarwal B, et al. Prevalence and outcomes of unoperated patients with severe symptomatic mitral regurgitation and heart failure: comprehensive analysis to determine the potential role of MitraClip for this unmet need. J Am Coll Cardiol 2014;63:185–6.

32. Silvestry FE, Rodriguez LL, Herrmann HC, et al. Echocardiographic guidance and assessment of percutaneous repair for mitral regurgitation with the Evalve MitraClip: lessons learned from EVERESTI. J Am Soc Echocardiogr 2007;20: 1131–40.

33. Lim DS, Reynolds MR, Feldman T, et al. Improved functional status and quality of life in prohibitive surgical risk patients with degenerative mitral regurgitation after transcatheter mitral valve repair. J Am Coll Cardiol 2014;64:182–92.

34. Sorajja P, Vemulapalli S, Feldman T, et al. Outcomes with transcatheter mitral valve repair in the United States: an STS/ACC TVT Registry report. J Am Coll Cardiol 2017;70:2315–27.

35. Lim, et al. Global EXPAND MitraClip Study. Poster presented at American College of Cardiology Conference. 2020.

A Review of the Partner Trials

Ryan Markham, MBBS, FRACP[a,b], Rahul Sharma, MBBS, FRACP[a,b],*

KEYWORDS

- Aortic stenosis • TAVR • PARTNER • Sapien heart valve • Clinical trial
- Aortic valve replacement

KEY POINTS

- Transcatheter aortic valve replacement (TAVR) has revolutionized the management of aortic stenosis (AS), with upward of 60,000 procedures being performed each year in the United States alone, outpacing the number of surgical aortic valve replacement procedures.
- The rapid uptake of TAVR technology and subsequent impact on clinical care was made possible due to the incredible body of evidence supporting the implementation of TAVR in high-risk, then intermediate-risk, and now low-risk patients.
- The PARTNER (Placement of Aortic Transcatheter Valves) trials were pivotal in presenting robust evidence for the safety, feasibility, and efficacy of TAVR in the management of AS and paved the way for clinical use worldwide.

INTRODUCTION

Aortic stenosis (AS) of moderate or greater severity has an estimated prevalence of 5% in people older than 65 years.[1] Survival is poor after onset of symptoms, and surgical aortic valve replacement (SAVR) was the gold-standard treatment for decades.[2] However, more than one-third of patients with symptomatic AS were untreated due to high surgical risk, exposing a clinical need for a less invasive therapy for aortic valve stenosis.[3] Balloon aortic valvuloplasty was the first nonsurgical therapy for this untreated patient cohort. However, the high restenosis rates following valvuloplasty failed to significantly change the natural history of AS and rendered the procedure palliative.[4] In April 2002, the first percutaneous implantation of an aortic valve bioprosthesis in a human was performed by Alain Cribier in a severely ill man with critical, calcific AS.[5] This marked the birth of transcatheter aortic valve replacement (TAVR). Since then, TAVR has revolutionized the management of AS, with upward of 60,000

procedures performed each year in the United States alone, outpacing the number of SAVR procedures.[6] The rapid uptake of TAVR technology and subsequent impact on clinical care was made possible due to the incredible body of evidence supporting the adoption of TAVR in high-risk, then intermediate-risk, and finally low-risk patients.[7] The PARTNER (Placement of Aortic Transcatheter Valves) trials were pivotal in presenting robust evidence for the safety, feasibility, and efficacy of TAVR in the management of AS and paved the way for its clinical use worldwide.

Partner 1B

The PARTNER 1B trial was a multicenter, randomized clinical trial comparing TAVR with standard therapy in high-risk patients with severe AS.[8] Severe AS was defined as a valve area less than or equal to 0.8 cm^2, mean aortic valve gradient greater than or equal to 40 mm Hg or more, or a peak aortic-jet velocity greater than or equal to 4.0 m per second with New York Heart Association (NYHA) class II, III, or IV

---

[a] Stanford Hospital, Palo Alto, CA, USA; [b] Department of Cardiovascular Medicine, Stanford Hospital, 300 Pasteur Drive, Room H2103, Stanford, CA 94305, USA
* Corresponding author. Department of Cardiovascular Medicine, Stanford Hospital, 300 Pasteur Drive, Room H2103, Stanford, CA 94305.
E-mail address: rpsharma@stanford.edu

Intervent Cardiol Clin 9 (2020) 461–467
https://doi.org/10.1016/j.iccl.2020.07.002
2211-7458/20/© 2020 Elsevier Inc. All rights reserved.

symptoms. Patients were divided into 2 cohorts: those who were considered to be candidates for surgery despite high surgical risk defined as a Society of Thoracic Surgeons (STS) risk score greater than or equal to 10% and those who were not considered suitable candidates for surgery due to coexisting conditions that would be associated with a predicted probability greater than or equal to 50% of either death at 30 days after surgery or a serious irreversible condition (Fig. 1).

Exclusion criteria included bicuspid AS, coronary artery disease needing revascularization, left ventricular ejection fraction less than 20%, severe mitral or aortic regurgitation, and transient ischemic attack or stroke within the prior 6 months of the procedure.

The Edwards SAPIEN heart valve system was used for the procedure. Valves were composed of bovine pericardium mounted in a balloon expandable stainless-steel frame, which were either 23 mm or 26 mm in diameter. The patient

was placed under general anesthesia and transesophageal echocardiography guidance was used. Balloon aortic valvuloplasty was performed followed by transfemoral insertion of a 22- or 24-French delivery sheath depending on the device size. The bioprosthetic valve was crimped onto a balloon catheter and advanced across the native aortic valve. Under rapid ventricular pacing via a temporary wire in the right ventricle, the balloon was inflated thereby expanding the frame and securing the valve to the native annular calcium. Patients were anticoagulated with heparin during the procedure and received dual antiplatelet therapy for 6 month following the procedure.

The primary endpoint was the rate of death from any cause over a follow-up period of 12 month. Prespecified secondary end points included the rate of death from cardiovascular causes, NYHA functional class, the rate of repeat hospitalization due to valve or procedure-related

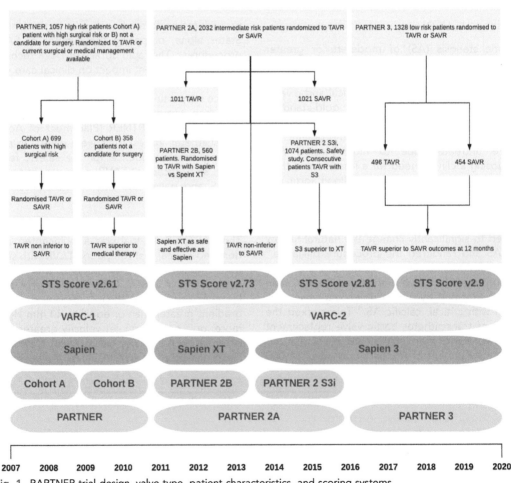

Fig. 1. PARTNER trial design, valve type, patient characteristics, and scoring systems.

clinical deterioration, myocardial infarction, acute kidney injury, and vascular complications.

A total of 358 patients were enrolled in the study, 179 receiving TAVR and 179 receiving standard therapy. The baseline characteristics were largely equivalent between both groups: mean STS score 12%, mean age 83 years, and aortic valve area 0.6 cm^2. Procedural outcomes were measured within the first 24 hours after the procedure during which 2 patients (1.1%) died and 3 (1.7%) suffered a stroke. At 30 days the rate of death from any cause was not significantly higher in the TAVR compared with standard therapy group (5% vs 2.8%, P = .41). However, at 1 year the rate of death was significantly lower in TAVR compared with standard therapy group (30.7% vs 50.7%, $P<.001$). The rate of cardiovascular death was also lower (20.5% vs 44.6%, $P<.001$). There were more major strokes in the TAVR group at 1 year (7.8% vs 3.9%, P = .18). The proportion of patients with no or mild dyspnea at 1 ear was also higher in patients who received TAVR (74.8% vs 40.0%, $P<.001$). Mean aortic valve area increased from 0.6 cm^2 to 1.5 cm^2 and mean aortic valve gradient decreased from 44.5% to 11.1% at 30 days, and these parameters were maintained out to 1-year.

It was concluded that in patients with severe AS who were not suitable candidates for surgery, TAVR as compared with standard therapy significantly reduced the rates of death from any cause and cardiovascular death at 1 year. This study paved the way for clinicians to utilize TAVR in the management of inoperable patients with severe AS who were previously only treated with medical therapy. Furthermore, it set the stage to test TAVR against SAVR in patients who were operable, albeit deemed high risk.

Partner 1A

In the PARTNER 1A trial 699 patients with severe AS underwent TAVR via transfemoral or transapical approach or SAVR.[9] Patients were those deemed to be at high risk for operative complications or death with SAVR. Inclusion and exclusion criteria were similar to those described in the PARTNER 1B trial. Primary outcome was death from any cause at 1 year, and prespecified secondary endpoints were similar to those described in the PARTNER 1A trial. Two hundred forty-four patients underwent transfemoral placement, 104 transapical placement, and 351 surgical placement (see **Fig. 1**). At 1 year the rate of death from any cause was 24.2% in the TAVR group and 26.8% in the SAVR group (P = .44 for superiority and P = .001 for

noninferiority). The rates of neurologic events were higher in the TAVR compared with SAVR group at 1 year (8.3% vs 4.3%, P = .04). From this the investigators concluded that TAVR was a reasonable alternative to SAVR in subgroup of patients with AS and high operative risk.

Having now established superiority to medical therapy in PARTNER B and equivalence to SAVR for select high-risk patients in PARTNER A, the next intuitive step was to compare TAVR with SAVR in intermediate risk patients who were candidates for SAVR.

Partner 2

Having established use in patients at high-risk for complications with SAVR, attention was then turned to intermediate-risk patients in the PARTNER 2A trial.[10] Two thousand thirty-two intermediate-risk patients with severe AS were assigned to undergo TAVR or SAVR (see **Fig. 1**). Intermediate risk was defined as an STS score greater than 4% and less than 8% although the upper limit was not prespecified. A newer generation, Sapien XT valve was used in this trial (https://www.edwards.com/devices/heart-valve s/sapien-xt-valve). Major differences between the Sapient XT and the Sapien valves included a thinner strut cobalt-chromium frame, partially closed resting valve leaflet geometry, reduced profile delivery system, and the addition of a 29 mm valve size option.[11]

The primary end point was death from any cause or disabling stroke at 2 years. A total of 1011 patients underwent TAVR and 1021 patients underwent SAVR. The mean STS score was 5.8% and mean age was 82 years in each group. There was no significant difference in the primary endpoint of death from any cause or stroke or disabling stroke at 2 years between the TAVR group and SAVR group (hazard ratio in the TAVR group: 0.89; 95% confidence interval, 0.73–1.09, P = .25). At 2 years these trends continued with rate of death and disabling stroke at 16.7% and 6.2% in the TAVR group and 18% and 6.4% in the SAVR group. Similar trends were seen in the transfemoral access subgroup but did not reach statistical significance. The investigators concluded that in intermediate-risk patients with severe symptomatic AS, SAVR, and TAVR resulted in no significant difference in the rates of death from any cause or disabling stroke and resulted in similar improvements in dyspnea.

This study opened the way for evaluating the use of TAVR in lower risk groups. However, the 6.4% risk of stroke associated with TAVR remained a concern, particularly as a potentially younger group of patients was to be considered for the procedure, and this led to heightened interest in the role of cerebral embolic protection devices with the goal of reduction in periprocedural strokes.[12–14]

Partner 3

The PARTNER 3 trial sought to evaluate TAVR versus SAVR in low-risk patients.[15] Patients with severe AS who were considered to be at low surgical risk were randomly assigned to undergo transfemoral TAVR or surgery. A newer generation Sapien 3 valve (Edwards Lifesciences, Irvine, CA) was used (https://www.edwards. com/devices/heart-valves/transcatheter-Sapien-3). The key development feature of the Sapein 3 valve is a polyethylene terephthalate fabric skirt on the distal section of the frame for prevention of paravalvular leak, which was a major limitation of earlier device iterations and was associated with worse long-term outcome.

The composite primary endpoint was the rate of death, stroke, or rehospitalization at 1 year (see **Fig. 1**). Key secondary endpoints were stroke, death and stroke, new onset atrial fibrillation, and length of index hospitalization. A total of 1000 patients were enrolled in the trial, and baseline characteristics were similar between groups, with a mean age of 73 years and mean STS score of 1.9%. The man aortic valve area was 0.8 cm^2 and mean aortic valve gradient was 49 mm Hg.

The primary endpoint was significantly lower in the TAVR compared with SAVR group (8.5% vs 15.1%, $P<.001$ for superiority). TAVR was also superior with regard to secondary endpoints, with lower rates of stroke (0.6% vs 2.4%, $P = .02$), death and stroke (1.0% vs 3.3%, $P = .01$), and new onset atrial fibrillation (5.0% vs 39.5%, $P<.001$).

Valve performance was equivalent between groups with mean aortic valve gradient 12.8 mm Hg in the TAVR group and 11.2 mm Hg in the SAVR group. The percentage of patients with moderate or severe paravalvular regurgitation did not differ significantly between the TAVR group and the surgery group (0.8% vs 0% respectively).

DISCUSSION

Over the past decade the use of TAVR in patients with severe, symptomatic AS has incrementally progressed from high to low surgical risk patients in concert with the results of the PARTNER trials. As valve technology has improved along with operator experience, the rates of procedural complications have decreased. Rates of death, stroke, vascular complications, need for pacemaker, and moderate or severe paravalvular regurgitation have declined significantly in the TAVR population over the past decade of PARTNER trials (**Fig. 2A–D**).

TAVR outcome reporting changed during the progression of the PARTNER trials (see **Fig. 1**). TAVR outcomes reporting was standardized with the Valve Academic Research Consortium (VARC) consensus document.[16] However, some definitions were ambiguous of limited clinical utility or required updating/extension. Notable changes included the need for risk stratification to be performed by a dedicated "heart team" and include other factors such as frailty and porcelain aorta, beyond the traditional risk score elements. Immediate procedural death was added to capture procedural events that led to immediate or consequent death. Stroke events were recategorized as disabling or nondisabling, and the cause of stroke was documented to help categorize as acute, early, or late stroke. Closure device failure was deemed a separate category within vascular complications. If an unplanned percutaneous or surgical procedure did not lead to an adverse outcome it was not considered as a major vascular complication. New definitions for several TAVR-related complications and valve malposition were also reported. Changes in quality-of-life measurements were implemented. These were largely incorporated in order to address the needs of future clinical trials and described in the VARC-2 consensus document.[17] The effects were analyzed in a retrospective study, which found that the VARC-2 definition of complications offered a better predictive value of survival than the VARC-1 definition.[18]

STS scoring systems also changed during the progression of the PARTNER trials (see **Fig. 1**). Overall, there was a general downward trend in absolute score—the same patient would have a lower calculated STS score with each updated version of the STS scoring system.[19] As a result, the use of current risk scores to stratify patients for TAVR or SAVR may not allow accurate comparison to patients in whom a differing STS risk calculator was used.[20] Despite updates to the STS score, there remain elements that contribute to overall risk not captured through the scoring system. The role of a cohesive "heart team" approach with interventional cardiologists, cardiothoracic surgeons, general physicians, imaging specialists, and allied health cannot be overstated.

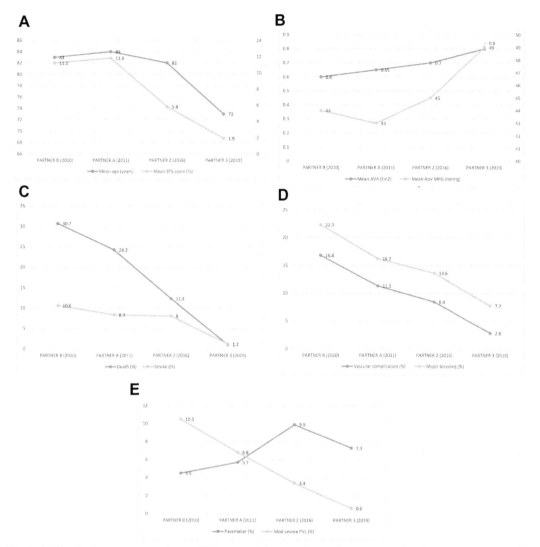

Fig. 2. (A) Decline in mean age and mean STS score. (B) Increase in baseline mean aortic valve area and aortic valve mean pressure gradient. (C) Decline in rates of death and stroke at 12 months. (D) Decline in rates of vascular complication and major bleeding. (E) Decline in rates of paravalvular leak with overall stable rates of new pacemaker postprocedure.

Around 60,000 TAVR procedures are performed annually in the United States, far outnumbering SAVR.[21] Two-thirds of these procedures are performed with the Edwards balloon expandable devices evaluated in the PARTNER trials. With the recent success of the PARTNER 3 trial, it is expected that the rates of TAVR utilization as a first-line therapy in younger, low-risk patients will increase overall TAVR volume.[22]

Despite the success of TAVR therapy thus far, there remain challenges and areas of uncertainty. The issue of subclinical and clinical valve thrombosis has been increasingly recognized, with a reported incidence between 7% and 14%.[23] The impact of this phenomenon on long-term valve durability becomes increasingly important, given the expansion of TAVR to low-risk patients. Surgical bioprosthetic valve durability is usually around 10 years.[24] Although 5-year durability results have been favorable for TAVR, the effect of leaflet crimping, balloon postdilatation, leaflet stress due to stent under-/overexpansion, and leaflet thrombosis/thickening in severely calcified aortic valves will only become clearer over a longer period of observation.[22]

The role of TAVR in aortic pathology outside of degenerative, calcific AS in a tricuspid valve is the subject of ongoing investigation. Bicuspid aortic valve disease is present in 2% of the population and comprises a clinically relevant proportion of patients referred for aortic valve intervention, particularly in a younger, low-risk cohort.[25] Several registries exist to assess the efficacy of TAVR in this population, and matched analyses have been performed to compare TAVR with surgery in bicuspid versus tricuspid aortic valves. The focus of these studies relate to the potential challenges and limitations of TAVR in bicuspid valves, including paravalvular leak, annular rupture, conduction disturbance, and stroke.[26,27]

The role of TAVR in patients with moderate AS with reduced left ventricular ejection fraction and in patients with asymptomatic, severe AS are currently the focus on clinical trials.[28] TAVR has been used in an off-label manner to treat pathologies involving the pulmonic, mitral, and tricuspid valves with varying degrees of success. Finally, the application of TAVR in aortic regurgitation is an ongoing area of interest.[29]

SUMMARY

Over the past decade the PARTNER trials have paved the way for the widespread use of TAVR in patients with severe, symptomatic AS stenosis. The role of the PARTNER trials in the evolution of TAVR cannot be overstated. The data from each of the trials have led, in a stepwise fashion, to the gradual and widespread adoption of a truly disruptive technology that continues to change the lives of patients, in whom surgery was previously the only possible solution. Underpinned by robust clinical evidence, the state of TAVR in contemporary clinical practice is the culmination of an orchestrated, multifaceted approach between physicians, engineers, industry, regulators, and ultimately, and most importantly, patients.

DISCLOSURE

Dr Rahul Sharma is a consultant and clinical proctor for Edwards Lifesciences.

REFERENCES

1. Nkomo VT, Gardin JM, Skelton TN, et al. Burden of valvular heart diseases: a population-based study. Lancet 2006;368(9540):1005–11.
2. Ross J Jr, Braunwald E. Aortic stenosis. Circulation 1968;38(1 Suppl):61–7.
3. Bach DS, Siao D, Girard SE, et al. Evaluation of patients with severe symptomatic aortic stenosis who do not undergo aortic valve replacement: the potential role of subjectively overestimated operative risk. Circ Cardiovasc Qual Outcomes 2009;2(6):533–9.
4. O'Neill WW. Predictors of long-term survival after percutaneous aortic valvuloplasty: report of the Mansfield Scientific Balloon Aortic Valvuloplasty Registry. J Am Coll Cardiol 1991;17(1):193–8.
5. Cribier A, Eltchaninoff H, Bash A, et al. Percutaneous transcatheter implantation of an aortic valve prosthesis for calcific aortic stenosis: first human case description. Circulation 2002;106(24):3006–8.
6. STS/ACC Registry data. Available at: https://www.sts.org/sites/default/files/102419%201645.%20Bavaria.%20TVT.pdf. Accessed April 28, 2020.
7. Cribier AG. The Odyssey of TAVR from concept to clinical reality. Tex Heart Inst J 2014;41(2):125–30.
8. Leon MB, Smith CR, Mack M, et al. Transcatheter aortic-valve implantation for aortic stenosis in patients who cannot undergo surgery. N Engl J Med 2010;363(17):1597–607.
9. Smith CR, Leon MB, Mack MJ, et al. Transcatheter versus surgical aortic-valve replacement in high-risk patients. N Engl J Med 2011;364(23):2187–98.
10. Leon MB, Smith CR, Mack MJ, et al. Transcatheter or surgical aortic-valve replacement in intermediate-risk patients. N Engl J Med 2016;374(17):1609–20.
11. Webb JG, Altwegg L, Masson JB, et al. A new transcatheter aortic valve and percutaneous valve delivery system. J Am Coll Cardiol 2009;53(20):1855–8.
12. Samim M, van der Worp B, Agostoni P, et al. TriGuard ™ HDH embolic deflection device for cerebral protection during transcatheter aortic valve replacement. Catheter Cardiovasc Interv 2017;89(3):470–7.
13. Latib A, Mangieri A, Vezzulli P, et al. First-in-man study evaluating the emblok embolic protection system during transcatheter aortic valve replacement. JACC Cardiovasc Interv 2020;13(7):860–8.
14. Schafer U. Safety and efficacy of protected cardiac intervention: clinical evidence for sentinel cerebral embolic protection. Interv Cardiol 2017;12(2):128–32.
15. Mack MJ, Leon MB, Thourani VH, et al. Transcatheter aortic-valve replacement with a balloon-expandable valve in low-risk patients. N Engl J Med 2019;380(18):1695–705.
16. Leon MB, Piazza N, Nikolsky E, et al. Standardized endpoint definitions for transcatheter aortic valve implantation clinical trials: a consensus report from the Valve Academic Research Consortium. J Am Coll Cardiol 2011;57(3):253–69.
17. Kappetein AP, Head SJ, Genereux P, et al. Updated standardized endpoint definitions for transcatheter aortic valve implantation: the Valve Academic Research Consortium-2 consensus document. J Am Coll Cardiol 2012;60(15):1438–54.

18. Okuyama K, Jilaihawi H, Abramowitz Y, et al. The clinical impact of vascular complications as defined by VARC-1 vs. VARC-2 in patients following transcatheter aortic valve implantation. Eurointervention 2016;12(5):e636–42.
19. Rogers T, Koifman E, Patel N, et al. Society of thoracic surgeons score variance results in risk reclassification of patients undergoing transcatheter aortic valve replacement. JAMA Cardiol 2017;2(4):455–6.
20. Kumar A, Sato K, Narayanswami J, et al. Current society of thoracic surgeons model reclassifies mortality risk in patients undergoing transcatheter aortic valve replacement. Circ Cardiovasc Interv 2018;11(9):e006664.
21. Grover FL, Vemulapalli S, Carroll JD, et al. 2016 annual report of the Society of Thoracic Surgeons/American College of Cardiology transcatheter valve therapy registry. Ann Thorac Surg 2017; 103(3):1021–35.
22. Boskovski MT, Nguyen TC, McCabe JM, et al. Outcomes of transcatheter aortic valve replacement in patients with severe aortic stenosis: a review of a disruptive technology in aortic valve surgery. JAMA Surg 2019 [Online ahead of print].
23. Hansson NC, Grove EL, Andersen HR, et al. Transcatheter aortic valve thrombosis: incidence, predisposing factors, and clinical implications. J Am Coll Cardiol 2016;68(19):2059–69.
24. Foroutan F, Guyatt GH, O'Brien K, et al. Prognosis after surgical replacement with a bioprosthetic aortic valve in patients with severe symptomatic aortic stenosis: systematic review of observational studies. BMJ 2016;354:i5065.
25. Michelena HI, Prakash SK, Della Corte A, et al. Bicuspid aortic valve: identifying knowledge gaps and rising to the challenge from the International Bicuspid Aortic Valve Consortium (BAVCon). Circulation 2014;129(25):2691–704.
26. Yoon SH, Sharma R, Chakravarty T, et al. Transcatheter aortic valve replacement in bicuspid aortic valve stenosis: where do we stand? J Cardiovasc Surg (Torino) 2018;59(3):381–91.
27. Yoon SH, Makkar R. Transcatheter aortic valve replacement for bicuspid aortic valve: challenges and pitfalls. Interv Cardiol Clin 2018; 7(4):477–88.
28. Rahhab Z, El Faquir N, Tchetche D, et al. Expanding the indications for transcatheter aortic valve implantation. Nat Rev Cardiol 2020;17(2):75–84.
29. Arias EA, Bhan A, Lim ZY, et al. TAVI for pure native aortic regurgitation: are we there yet? Interv Cardiol 2019;14(1):26–30.

COURAGE, ORBITA, and ISCHEMIA

Percutaneous Coronary Intervention for Stable Coronary Artery Disease

Zhi Teoh, MA, MBBChir, MRCP[a],
Rasha K. Al-Lamee, MA, MB BS, MRCP, PhD[b,c,*]

KEYWORDS

- Percutaneous coronary intervention • Angina • Ischemia • Placebo
- Chronic coronary artery disease

KEY POINTS

- Percutaneous coronary intervention (PCI) in stable coronary artery disease (CAD) has not been shown to improve mortality or overall myocardial infarction (MI) rates.
- Rather, risk reduction with medical therapy remains the most important intervention for reducing mortality and MI rate.
- The primary indication of PCI in stable CAD remains symptom relief.
- The role of placebo in symptom relief, however, may be underestimated. Placebo-controlled trials are needed to quantify the true physiologic effect of PCI.
- Even in the presence of significant ischemia, an invasive treatment has not been proved to be superior to conservative treatment in improving outcomes.

INTRODUCTION

Four decades ago, percutaneous coronary intervention (PCI) was first introduced to treat angina in stable coronary artery disease (CAD).[1] Today, more than 500,000 PCI procedures are performed annually, primarily for this indication.[2]

This review article aims to summarize some of the key trials that have shaped understanding of the role of PCI in stable CAD.

PERCUTANEOUS CORONARY INTERVENTION FOR SYMPTOM RELIEF

It is widely accepted that angina results from inadequate myocardial perfusion. Therefore, it seems intuitive that, in patients who present with angina and are found to have reduced myocardial perfusion due to an epicardial stenosis, resolution of the stenosis with PCI may improve angina. In unblinded trials of stable CAD—Study of Angioplasty Compared to Medical Therapy (ACME), Clinical Outcomes Utilizing Revascularization and Aggressive Drug Evaluation (COURAGE), Fractional Flow Reserve–guided PCI versus Medical Therapy in Stable Coronary Disease (FAME 2), and International Study of Comparative Health Effectiveness with Medical and Invasive Approaches (ISCHEMIA)—significant improvement in angina and quality of life was seen with unblinded PCI.[3–6] More than one-third of patients, however, continued to have symptoms despite successful revascularization.[7–9]

[a] Barts Health NHS Trust, The Royal London Hospital, 80 Newark Street, London E1 2ES, UK; [b] Imperial College Healthcare NHS Trust, Hammersmith Hospital, Du Cane Road, London W12 0HS, UK; [c] Imperial College London, Hammersmith Hospital, Du Cane Road, London W12 0HS, UK
* Corresponding author. Imperial College Healthcare NHS Trust, Hammersmith Hospital, Du Cane Road, London W12 0HS, UK.
E-mail address: r.al-lamee13@imperial.ac.uk

2211-7458/20/© 2020 Elsevier Inc. All rights reserved.

Importantly, symptoms are subjective. In assessing the effect of any intervention on a subjective endpoint, the presence of both a true physiologic effect and a placebo component must be acknowledged. The placebo component is larger with invasive than noninvasive treatments. Blinding is required to quantify the true physiologic effect size beyond placebo. In unblinded trials of stable CAD, patients and physicians were aware of treatment allocation. Placebo-controlled symptom relief, therefore, was unknown. The first placebo-controlled trial of PCI, Objective Randomised Blinded Investigation with Optimal Medical Therapy of Angioplasty in Stable Angina (ORBITA), recruited patients with angiographically severe single-vessel disease.[10] After 6 weeks of medical optimization with risk prevention and antianginal medication, patients were randomized to PCI or a placebo procedure. They then entered a 6-week blinded follow-up phase. The primary endpoint was the difference in treadmill exercise time increment between the groups.

The majority of patients had severe single vessel coronary artery dise with mean area stenosis of 84.4% (SD 10.2), mean fractional flow reserve (FFR) 0.69 (SD 0.16), and mean instantaneous wave-free ratio (iFR) 0.76 (SD 0.22). For comparison, mean FFR was 0.71 (SD 0.18) and 0.68 (SD 0.10) in FAME and FAME 2, respectively.[3,11]

To the surprise of many, despite significant improvement in placebo-controlled stress echocardiography ischemia in the PCI arm, there was no detectable difference in exercise time increment between the PCI and placebo group. There also were no detectable differences in patient-reported or physician-assessed symptoms or quality of life. In a secondary analysis, the only symptom endpoint in which there was a between-group difference was the Seattle Angina Questionnaire freedom from angina, where PCI resulted in 1 in 5 more patients in the PCI arm were free from angina than the placebo arm.[12]

From unblinded data and unblinded clinical experience, is it possible that the impact of placebo on symptom relief was underestimated?

PERCUTANEOUS CORONARY INTERVENTION FOR MORTALITY IMPROVEMENT

Despite its initial remit for treating angina, it began to be assumed that PCI could achieve more than just symptom relief. It was suggested that PCI might reduce rates of death and myocardial infarction (MI).

Although PCI in the setting of acute coronary syndrome is certainly associated with a reduction in mortality and MI,[13-15] in stable CAD, its role for these endpoints is more controversial.

The COURAGE trial compared PCI to no PCI, with medical therapy given to both groups, in 2287 patients with stable CAD,[6] the primary outcome being death from any cause or nonfatal MI. The trial showed no difference in mortality or MI between both groups, a result that had been seen in other smaller previous trials (Table 1).

This result led to significant soul-searching among interventional cardiologists. Nonetheless, advocates for PCI felt that COURAGE had several limitations. First, a majority of patients in the PCI arm were treated with bare-metal stents because drug-eluting stents were not approved for clinical use until late in the trial. Second, a sizable proportion of the patients did not have significant ischemia, as demonstrated in the COURAGE nuclear substudy, which showed that two-thirds of patients had less than 10% ischemia on myocardial perfusion imaging.[16]

Exponents of this view refer to the FAME 2 trial, in which patients with significant coronary ischemia (as demonstrated by an FFR ≤0.8) were randomized to either PCI (with second-generation drug eluting stents) or no PCI.[3] In this study, the primary outcome, which was a composite of death, MI, and urgent revascularization, significantly favored the PCI group, with a 68% reduction in primary endpoint. The trial was halted early due to a highly significant incidence of urgent revascularization events in the no-PCI group. This outcome was driven primarily by increased rates of urgent revascularization, which in approximately 50% of these cases, were performed based on clinical symptoms alone with no ECG change or rise in cardiac biomarkers, an event that could have reflected the unblinded trial design.[17] Importantly, for endpoints less susceptible to issues with blinding, no significant difference in mortality or MI rates was observed.

Two years later, the FAME 2 investigators, by excluding the periprocedural events or early postprocedural events in the first 7 days from analysis, found that the PCI group had a lower rate of death or MI.[18] Yet, without this correction, even at 5 years, there was no significant difference in the individual outcomes of death or MI between the 2 groups.[19]

Table 1
Trials comparing percutaneous coronary intervention to conservative treatment

Trial	Inclusion Criteria	N	Follow-up	Description of Medical Therapy	Definition of Nonfatal Myocardial Infarction	ETT Protocol	Primary Endpoint	Primary Endpoint Result
[a]ACME, 1992[4]	Men with 1-VD (70%–99% stenosis with exercise-induced myocardial ischemia)	212	6 mo	Isosorbide dinitrate, nitroglycerin, β-blockers, CCB or a combination of these, increased as needed to maximum tolerated dose	New Q-waves or CK increase above normal limits, in combination with typical clinical signs	Modified Bruce	Change in exercise tolerance, frequency of angina attacks and use of nitroglycerin	Exercise time improved but no difference for other primary endpoints
[a]MASS, 1995[20]	Prox LAD only, >80% stenosis	144	3 y	β-Blockers, CCB, nitrates, aspirin	New Q-waves in at least 2 ECG leads or typical clinical symptoms with CK rise ≥3-times normal upper limit	Modified Bruce	Combined incidence of cardiac death, MI or refractory angina requiring revascularization	No difference
[a]ACME 2, 1997[21]	Men with 2-VD	328	6 mo	Aspirin plus nitrates, β-blockers, CCB in progressive stepped approach	New Q waves in any anterior or lateral lead or in 2 or more contiguous inferior leads on a follow-up ECG or hospital admission for chest pain accompanied by serum enzyme changes meeting local hospital criteria for MI	Modified Bruce	Angina frequency, freedom from angina, exercise time, change in angiographic stenosis	No difference

(continued on next page)

Trial	Inclusion Criteria	N	Follow-up	Description of Medical Therapy	Definition of Nonfatal Myocardial Infarction	ETT Protocol	Primary Endpoint	Primary Endpoint Result
[a]RITA-2, 1997[22]	≥1-VD	1018	2.7 y (median)	β-Blockers, CCB, long-acting nitrates	New Q-waves on ECG or convincing clinical history associated with ECG changes compatible with non-Q wave infarction and serum activities ≥2 cardiac enzymes were above 2-times upper limit of normal	Full Bruce	All-cause death and nonfatal MI	Increased risk of death and MI in PCI group
[a]ACME extended follow-up, 1998[23]	Provocable myocardial ischemia and 1-VD >70%	212	3 y	N/A	New Q-waves or CK increase above normal limits, in combination with typical clinical signs	Modified Bruce	N/A	N/A
AVERT, 1999[24]	Stable CAD with ≥1-VD, asymptomatic or mild-to-moderate angina	341	18 mo	Atorvastatin, 80 mg on	N/A	Full Bruce	Combined outcome of death from cardiac causes, resuscitation after cardiac arrest, non-fatal MI, cerebrovascular accident, CABG, angioplasty, or worsening angina with objective evidence resulting in hospitalization	Reduction of primary outcome in PCI group but not statistically significant

Trial	Inclusion	N	Follow-up	Medical therapy	MI definition	Exercise test	Primary endpoint	Result
DEFER, 2001[25]	1-VD and FFR ≥0.75	181	2 y	Deferral	Pathologic Q waves on ECG or an increase of serum CK levels to more than twice the normal value	N/A	Absence of all-cause mortality, MI, CABG, coronary angioplasty, any procedure-related complication necessitating major intervention	No difference
RITA-2 7-y follow-up, 2003[26]	≥1-VD	1018	7 y (median)	β-Blockers, CCB, long-acting nitrates	New Q-waves on ECG or convincing clinical history associated with ECG changes compatible with non-Q wave infarction and serum activities ≥2 cardiac enzymes were above 2 times upper limit of normal	Full Bruce	Death and MI	No difference
MASS II, 2004[27]	Prox 2-VD/3-VD/LAD disease	408	5 y	Nitrates, β-blockers, CCB, ACE inhibitors, aspirin, statins	New Q-waves in at least 2 ECG leads or typical clinical symptoms with CK rise ≥3 times normal upper limit	Modified Bruce	Combined incidence of cardiac death, MI, or refractory angina requiring revascularization	Significant increase of primary event in PCI group (driven by need for additional revascularization procedures)

(continued on next page)

Trial	Inclusion Criteria	N	Follow-up	Description of Medical Therapy	Definition of Nonfatal Myocardial Infarction	ETT Protocol	Primary Endpoint	Primary Endpoint Result
COURAGE, 2007[6]	Stable CAD, 1-VD, 2-VD, or 3-VD	2287	4.6 y (median)	Aspirin and clopidogrel, long-acting metoprolol, amlodipine and isosorbide mononitrate alone or in combination, along with either lisinopril or losartan	Clinical presentation consistent with ACS and either new abnormal Q-waves in $\geq$2 ECG leads or positive results in cardiac biomarkers, OR abnormal Q waves alone (silent MI)	N/A	Composite all-cause death and nonfatal MI	No difference
JSAP, 2008[28]	1-VD or 2-VD	384	3 y	Antianginals and risk factor modification	New abnormal Q-waves in $\geq$2 ECG leads or convincing clinical history with ECG compatible with non–Q-wave infarction and serum activities of $\geq$2 cardiac enzymes greater than twice normal	N/A	Death, ACS, CVA or emergency hospitalization	Reduction in primary outcome in PCI group (driven by reduction in unstable angina)

COURAGE, ORBITA, and ISCHEMIA 475

BARI-2D, 2009[29]	T2DM with stable IHD	1605	5.3 y	Based on current guidelines for lipid and blood pressure management, smoking cessation, physical activity, and weight loss	Abnormal biomarker profile ≥ twice upper limits of normal and evidence of angina or angina-equivalent symptoms, ECG or imaging evidence of new MI	N/A	All-cause death, cardiac death, MI	No difference
MASS II extended follow-up, 2010[30]	Proximal 2-VD/3-VD/LAD disease	408	10 y	Nitrates, β-blockers, CCB, ACE inhibitors, Aspirin, statins	New Q-waves in at least 2 ECG leads or typical clinical symptoms with CK rise ≥3-times normal upper limit	Modified Bruce	Combined incidence of all-cause mortality, Q-wave MI, or refractory angina requiring revascularization	No significant difference between PCI and medical therapy group
FAME II, 2012[3]	1-VD, 2-VD, or 3-VD and FFR ≤0.8	888	213 d (mean)	β-Blockers, CCB, long-acting nitrates, lisinopril, aspirin, atorvastatin	N/A	N/A	Composite of death, nonfatal MI, or urgent revascularization	Reduction of primary outcome in PCI group (driven by urgent revascularization)

(continued on next page)

Trial	Inclusion Criteria	N	Follow-up	Description of Medical Therapy	Definition of Nonfatal Myocardial Infarction	ETT Protocol	Primary Endpoint	Primary Endpoint Result
COURAGE extended follow-up, 2015[31]	Stable CAD, 1-VD, 2-VD, or 3-VD	1211	15 y	Aspirin and clopidogrel, long-acting metoprolol, amlodipine and isosorbide mononitrate alone or in combination, along with either lisinopril or losartan	N/A	N/A	Death	No difference (32.6% crossover)
DEFER extended follow-up, 2015[32]	1-VD and FFR ≥0.75	N/A	15 y	Deferral	Pathologic Q waves on ECG or an increase of serum CK-levels to more than twice the normal value	N/A	Death, MI or repeat revascularization	Higher rate of MI observed in PCI group. No difference observed in mortality or rate of repeat revascularization[b]
ORBITA, 2018[10]	1-VD	200	6 wk	Intensive up-titration of antianginals	N/A	Modified Bruce	Exercise time increment between groups	No difference
FAME II extended follow-up, 2018[19]	1-VD, 2-VD, or 3-VD and FFR ≤0.8	888	5 y	β-Blockers, CCB, long-acting nitrates, lisinopril, aspirin, atorvastatin	N/A	N/A	Composite of death, MI, or urgent revascularization	Reduction of primary outcome in PCI group (driven by urgent revascularization)

| ISCHEMIA, 2020[5] | Stable IHD and moderate-to-severe ischemia on noninvasive stress testing | 5179 | 3.2 y[c] | Antiplatelets, statin, other lipid-lowering, antihypert-ensives and anti-ischemic medical therapies, diet, physical activity, and smoking cessation | Clinical setting consistent with ACS with troponin elevation above upper limit of normal and at least: Symptoms of ischemia >20mins/New ischemic ECG changes, Q waves or LBBB/Imaging evidence of new loss of viable myocardium/ Angiographic evidence of intracoronary thrombus, stent thrombosis or high-grade in-stent restenosis | N/A | Composite of cardiovascular death, MI, resuscitated cardiac arrest, or hospitalization for unstable angina/ heart failure | No difference |

Abbreviations: ACE, angiotensin converting enzyme inhibitors; ACS, acute coronary syndrome; CCB, calcium channel blockers; CK, creatinine kinase; ECG, electrocardiogram; ETT, exercise tolerance test; IHD, ischemic heart disease; LAD, left anterior descending artery; T2DM, type 2 diabetes mellitus; VD, vessel disease.

[a] Plain balloon angioplasty.
[b] Not powered for 15-y follow-up.
[c] Invasive arm including revascularization with PCI or CABG.

Table 2
Clinical events in trials comparing percutaneous coronary intervention to conservative treatment

Trial	n Percutaneous Coronary Intervention	n No Percutaneous Coronary Intervention	Nonfatal Myocardial Infarction — Percutaneous Coronary Intervention	No Percutaneous Coronary Intervention	P Value	Cardiac Death — Percutaneous Coronary Intervention	No Percutaneous Coronary Intervention	P Value	All-Cause Mortality — Percutaneous Coronary Intervention	No Percutaneous Coronary Intervention	P Value	Urgent/Repeat Revascularization — Percutaneous Coronary Intervention	No Percutaneous Coronary Intervention	P Value
ACME, 1992[4]	105	107	5 (4.8%)	3 (2.8%)	.5	0 (0%)	1 (0.9%)	1	0 (0%)	1 (0.9%)	1	16 (15.0%)	11 (10.3%)	N/A
MASS, 1995[20]	72	72	0 (0%)	2 (2.8%)	N/A	1 (1.4%)	0 (0%)	N/A	1 (1.4%)	0 (0%)	N/A	29 (40.3%)	7 (9.7%)	N/A
ACME 2, 1997[21]	166	162	2 (1.2%)	6 (3.7%)	N/A	N/A	N/A	N/A	2 (1.2%)	1 (0.6%)	N/A	11 (6.6%)	8 (4.9%)	N/A
RITA-2, 1997[22]	504	514	21 (4.2%)	10 (1.9%)	N/A	5 (1.0%)	3 (0.6%)	N/A	11 (2.2%)	7 (1.4%)	N/A	102 (20.2%)	131 (25.5%)	N/A
ACME extended follow-up, 1998[23]	105	107	10 (9.5%)	7 (6.5%)	N/A	N/A	N/A	N/A	5 (4.8%)	7 (6.5%)	.58	31 (35%)	34 (42%)	.72
AVERT, 1999[24]	177	164	5 (2.8%)	4 (2.4%)	N/A	1 (0.6%)	1 (0.6%)	N/A	N/A	N/A	N/A	21 (11.9%)	18 (11.0%)	N/A
DEFER, 2001[25]	90	91	1 (1.1%)	0 (0%)	N/A	1 (1.1%)	2 (2.2%)	N/A	2 (2.2%)	4 (4.4%)	N/A	10 (11.1%)	6 (6.6%)	N/A
RITA-2 7-y follow-up, 2003[26]	504	514	32 (6.3%)	23 (4.5%)	N/A	13 (2.6%)	22 (4.3%)	N/A	43 (8.5%)	43 (8.4%)	N/A	137 (27.2%)	182 (35.4%)	N/A
MASS II, 2004[27]	205	203	16 (8%)	10 (5%)	N/A	9 (4.5%)	3 (1.5%)	N/A	9 (4.5%)	3 (1.5%)	N/A	25 (12.2%)	16 (7.9%)	N/A
COURAGE, 2007[6]	1149	1138	143 (13.2%)	128 (12.3%)	.33	23 (2%)	25 (2.2%)	N/A	85 (7.6%)	95 (8.3%)	.38	228 (21.1%)	348 (32.6%)	.001
JSAP, 2008[28]	192	192	3 (1.6%)	7 (3.7%)	.2	2 (1%)	3 (1.6%)	N/A	6 (2.9%)	7 (3.9%)	.79	26.40%	48.50%	N/A
BARI-2D, 2009[29]	798	807	95 (12.3%)	88 (12.6%)	.42	44 (5%)	33 (4.2%)	.16	102 (10.8%)	96 (10.2%)	.48	315 (43.3%)	452 (42.1%)	N/A

Study														
MASS II extended follow-up, 2010[30]	205	203	13.30%	20.70%	n/a	14.30%	20.70%	N/A	24.10%	31.00%	N/A	41.90%	39.40%	N/A
FAME 2, 2012[3]	447	441	15 (3.4%)	14 (3.2%)	.89	1 (0.2%)	1 (0.2%)	.98	1 (0.2%)	3 (0.7%)	.31	14 (3.1%)	86 (19.5%)	<.001
COURAGE extended follow-up, 2015[31]	613	598	N/A	N/A	N/A	N/A	N/A	N/A	284 (25%)	277 (24%)	.76	N/A	N/A	N/A
DEFER extended follow-up, 2015[32]	90	91	9 (10%)	2 (2.2%)	.03	4 (4.4%)	5 (5.5%)	1	28 (31.1%)	30 (33%)	.79	31 (34.4%)	39 (42.9%)	.245
ORBITA, 2018[10]	105	95	N/A	N/A	N/A	N/A	N/A	N/A	0 (0%)	0 (0%)	N/A	0 (0%)	1 (1.1%)	N/A
FAME 2 extended follow-up, 2018[19]	447	441	36 (8.1%)	53 (12%)	N/A	11 (2.5%)	7 (1.6%)	No difference	23 (5.1%)	23 (5.2%)	no difference	60 (13.4%)	225 (51%)	Reduction in PCI group
ISCHEMIA, 2020[5]	N/A[a]	2591	N/A	N/A[b]	233 (9.0%)	N/A	N/A[c]	111 (4.3%)	N/A[d]	144 (5.6%)	N/A	N/A	N/A	N/A

[a] 2588 patients randomized to revascularization therapy, including either PCI or CABG. Only combined data available for PCI and CABG in invasive arm.
[b] 210 (8.1%) in revascularization group.
[c] 92 (3.6%) in revascularization group.
[d] 145 (5.6%) in revascularization group.

Table 2 summarizes the results of other RCTs examining mortality, MI, and urgent revascularization outcomes over the past few years.

One final question remained: Were the results of previous trials affected by inclusion of patients with too little ischemia and would revascularization lead to better outcomes if it was targeted to patients with the highest ischemic burden? ISCHEMIA trial was designed to answer this question; 5179 patients from 320 centers worldwide with moderate to severe ischemia on noninvasive stress testing were randomized prior to invasive coronary angiography to either an invasive or a conservative strategy, with medical therapy given to both groups. The primary outcome consisted of a composite of death, MI, resuscitated cardiac arrest, or hospitalization for unstable angina or heart failure. An invasive strategy, which consisted of invasive coronary angiography plus revascularization as appropriate with coronary artery bypass graft surgery (CABG) or PCI, did not prove superior to a conservative strategy in reducing the composite primary endpoint or the major secondary endpoint of death or MI.

In the invasive arm, there was a 1% absolute increase in periprocedural MIs (defined as MI in the first 6 months) followed by a 1% absolute decrease in spontaneous MIs (defined as MIs sustained 6 months after the initial procedure) within 4 years. The significance of this finding is difficult to understand in the short term because it did not result in any differences in cardiovascular death or urgent revascularization between the groups. Importantly, there was no difference in the overall MI rate between the groups. Long term follow-up from ISCHEMIA is needed to understand its true clinical implications.

PUTTING COURAGE, ORBITA, AND ISCHEMIA IN CONTEXT

Many investigators now question the place of revascularization in stable CAD now that there are data from these landmark trials. There are many implications for practice.

First, it must be remembered that the results apply only to the patients who were studied. The role of revascularization in patients who were excluded from the trials, for example, those with moderate to severe left ventricular dysfunction, left main stem disease, remains unknown.

For the remainder, the most important message must be that revascularization is unlikely to improve mortality or MI rates in the majority. This must be conveyed to patients and referring physicians who predominantly still believe that PCI saves lives in stable CAD. They must understand that the primary remit remains symptom relief.

In order to prevent death and MI, optimum event prevention and risk factor modification with medical therapy must be ensured in all patients with stable CAD. This step saves lives and changes long-term outcomes.

For symptom relief, it must be understood that placebo does have an influence and is undeniably part of medical care. Part of being a good medical practitioner is the ability to make patients feel safe, secure, and well looked after. In designing future trials of intervention with subjective endpoints, it is important to consider the necessity for placebo-controlled trial design to quantify the true physiologic effect of the treatment.

The results of these trials must be used in shared decision making with patients. Some patients always opt for an upfront procedure even if there is clinical equipoise. Others prefer to try medical therapy and prefer to avoid a procedure with possible short-term and long-term complications, if they can have event prevention and relief of symptoms with medical therapy alone.

The most important consideration is the value of ischemia. ORBITA has shown that the link between epicardial coronary stenosis, ischemia, and symptoms is more complex than was assumed. ISCHEMIA and COURAGE have shown that relief of ischemia does not have an impact on outcomes. Perhaps detection of ischemia is merely important in diagnosing CAD. The burden of ischemia is only a reflection of the burden of atherosclerosis and merely treating what is seen with revascularization does not change clinical outcomes because the intervention does not modify the underlying disease process. This calls into question the importance of silent ischemia or high ischemic burden and suggests that there may be no need for early revascularization in these patients. Additionally, there should be no role for the use of tests of ischemia for routine surveillance or to guide therapy in the majority of asymptomatic patients with good left ventricular systolic function and no significant left main disease.

SUMMARY

The relationship between stenosis, ischemia, and angina is more complex than first imagined. The primary remit of revascularization in stable CAD remains symptom relief, albeit with the caveat that some of this symptom relief may be the result of placebo. Detection of ischemia may continue to be important in the diagnosis of CAD but is not as useful as once considered in guiding treatment. For mortality and MI reduction, the most important intervention is adequate risk reduction medical therapy. Although the debate continues, it must be remembered that these trials should be used to educate and to guide shared decision making in patients with stable CAD.

DISCLOSURE

Dr Al-Lamee has received speaker's honoraria from Philips Volcano.

REFERENCES

1. Grüntzig A. Transluminal dilatation of coronary-artery stenosis. Lancet 1978;311(8058):263.
2. Brown DL, Redberg RF. Last nail in the coffin for PCI in stable angina? Lancet 2018;391(10115):3–4.
3. De Bruyne B, Pijls NHJ, Kalesan B, et al. Fractional flow reserve–guided PCI versus medical therapy in stable coronary disease. N Engl J Med 2012;367(11):991–1001.
4. Parisi AF, Folland ED, Hartigan P. A comparison of angioplasty with medical therapy in the treatment of single-vessel coronary artery disease. Veterans Affairs ACME Investigators. N Engl J Med 1992;326(1):10–6.
5. Maron DJ, Hochman JS, Reynolds HR, et al. Initial invasive or conservative strategy for stable coronary disease. N Engl J Med 2020;382(15):1395-407.
6. Boden WE, O'Rourke RA, Teo KK, et al. Optimal medical therapy with or without PCI for stable coronary disease. N Engl J Med 2007;356(15):1503–16.
7. Dagenais GR, Lu J, Faxon DP, et al. Effects of optimal medical treatment with or without coronary revascularization on angina and subsequent revascularizations in patients with type 2 diabetes mellitus and stable ischemic heart disease. Circulation 2011;123(14):1492–500.
8. Niccoli G, Montone RA, Lanza GA, et al. Angina after percutaneous coronary intervention: The need for precision medicine. Int J Cardiol 2017;248:14–9.
9. Arnold SV, Jang J-S, Tang F, et al. Prediction of residual angina after percutaneous coronary intervention. Eur Heart J Qual Care Clin Outcomes 2015;1(1):23–30.
10. Al-Lamee R, Thompson D, Dehbi HM, et al. Percutaneous coronary intervention in stable angina (ORBITA): a double-blind, randomised controlled trial. Lancet 2018;391(10115):31–40.
11. Tonino PAL, De Bruyne B, Pijls NHJ, et al. Fractional flow reserve versus angiography for guiding percutaneous coronary intervention. N Engl J Med 2009;360(3):213–24.
12. Al-Lamee R, Howard JP, Shun-Shin MJ, et al. Fractional flow reserve and instantaneous wave-free ratio as predictors of the placebo-controlled response to percutaneous coronary intervention in stable single-vessel coronary artery disease. Circulation 2018;138(17):1780–92.
13. Weaver WD. Comparison of primary coronary angioplasty and intravenous thrombolytic therapy for acute myocardial infarction. JAMA 1997;278(23):2093.
14. Keeley EC, Boura JA, Grines CL. Primary angioplasty versus intravenous thrombolytic therapy for acute myocardial infarction: A quantitative review of 23 randomised trials. Lancet 2003;361(9351):13–20.
15. O'neill W, Timmis GC, Bourdillon PD, et al. A prospective randomized clinical trial of intracoronary streptokinase versus coronary angioplasty for acute myocardial infarction. N Engl J Med 1986;314(13):812–8.
16. Shaw LJ, Berman DS, Maron DJ, et al. Optimal medical therapy with or without percutaneous coronary intervention to reduce ischemic burden. Circulation 2008;117(10):1283–91.
17. Rajkumar CA, Nijjer SS, Cole GD, et al. Moving the goalposts into unblinded territory: the larger lessons of DEFER and FAME 2 and their implications for shifting end points in ISCHEMIA. Circ Cardiovasc Qual Outcomes 2018;11(3):e004665.
18. De Bruyne B, Fearon WF, Pijls NHJ, et al. Fractional flow reserve–guided pci for stable coronary artery disease. N Engl J Med 2014;371(13):1208–17.
19. Xaplanteris P, Fournier S, Pijls NHJ, et al. Five-year outcomes with pci guided by fractional flow reserve. N Engl J Med 2018;379(3):250–9.
20. Hueb WA, Bellotti G, de Oliveira SA, et al. The Medicine, Angioplasty or Surgery Study (MASS): A prospective, randomized trial of medical therapy, balloon angioplasty or bypass surgery for single proximal left anterior descending artery stenoses. J Am Coll Cardiol 1995;26(7):1600–5.
21. Folland ED, Hartigan PM, Parisi AF. Percutaneous transluminal coronary angioplasty versus medical therapy for stable angina pectoris: Outcomes for patients with double-vessel versus single-vessel coronary artery disease in a veterans affairs cooperative randomized trial. J Am Coll Cardiol 1997;29(7):1505–11.
22. Pocock S. Coronary angioplasty versus medical therapy for angina: The second randomised intervention treatment of angina (RITA-2) trial. Lancet 1997;350(9076):461–8.
23. Hartigan PM, Giacomini JC, Folland ED, et al. Two- to three-year follow-up of patients with single-vessel coronary artery disease randomized to

PTCA or medical therapy (Results of a VA cooperative study). Am J Cardiol 1998;82(12):1445–50.

24. Pitt B, Waters D, Brown WV, et al. Aggressive lipid-lowering therapy compared with angioplasty in stable coronary artery disease. N Engl J Med 1999; 341(2):70–6.

25. Bech GJW, De Bruyne B, Pijls NHJ, et al. Fractional flow reserve to determine the appropriateness of angioplasty in moderate coronary stenosis: A randomized trial. Circulation 2001;103(24):2928–34.

26. Henderson RA, Pocock SJ, Clayton TC, et al. Seven-year outcome in the RITA-2 trial: Coronary angioplasty versus medical therapy. J Am Coll Cardiol 2003;42(7):1161–70.

27. Hueb W, Soares PR, Gersh BJ, et al. The medicine, angioplasty, or surgery study (MASS-II): A randomized, controlled clinical trial of three therapeutic strategies for multivessel coronary artery disease: One-year results. J Am Coll Cardiol 2004;43(10): 1743–51.

28. Nishigaki K, Yamazaki T, Kitabatake A, et al. Percutaneous coronary intervention plus medical therapy reduces the incidence of acute coronary syndrome more effectively than initial medical therapy only among patients with low-risk coronary artery disease. a randomized, comparative, multicenter study. JACC Cardiovasc Interv 2008;1(5):469–79.

29. Frye RL, August P, Brooks MM, et al. A randomized trial of therapies for type 2 diabetes and coronary artery disease. N Engl J Med 2009;360(24):2503–15.

30. Hueb W, Lopes N, Gersh BJ, et al. Ten-year follow-up survival of the Medicine, Angioplasty, or Surgery Study (MASS II): a randomized controlled clinical trial of 3 therapeutic strategies for multivessel coronary artery disease. Circulation 2010;122(10):949–57.

31. Sedlis SP, Hartigan PM, Teo KK, et al. Effect of PCI on long-term survival in patients with stable ischemic heart disease. N Engl J Med 2015; 373(20):1937–46.

32. Zimmermann FM, Ferrara A, Johnson NP, et al. Deferral vs. performance of percutaneous coronary intervention of functionally non-significant coronary stenosis: 15-year follow-up of the DEFER trial. Eur Heart J 2015;36(45):3182–8.

Renal Denervation
History and Current Status

David P. Lee, MD

KEYWORDS

• Renal denervation • Hypertension • Catheter

KEY POINTS

- Review of the early history of renal denervation, including its conceptualization and early surgical experience as well as eventual catheter creation.
- Clinical trial and data regarding renal denervation are discussed with an examination of the early studies and their results as well as current clinical trials.
- Suggestions about the future direction of renal denervation and expansion into areas beyond hypertension.

INTRODUCTION

The worldwide incidence of hypertension (HTN) is approximately 30% and affects more than 1 billion people. For years, lifestyle management and medications have been the mainstay of therapy but medical compliance remains approximately 60% to 70% in developed countries. New and novel approaches to the treatment of HTN are important, and borne out of this need is the technique of catheter-based renal denervation (RDN). There have been some challenges in defining the most appropriate hypertensive population for RDN as well as the magnitude of benefit for this procedure.

BACKGROUND

The concept of RDN was borne out of seminal work in the 1940s by Smithwick and Thompson.[1] In their work, open surgical renal sympathectomy was performed in patients with refractory HTN, a reflection of the urgency for therapy in this era. Although open surgical sympathectomy worked to treated severe HTN and demonstrated a mortality benefit, the risk of the procedure as well as the side effects of hypotension and loss of appropriate sympathetic response led to dismissal of the technique by the late 1950s. In the early 2000s, Andrew Cleeland and others began to re-explore the concept of denervation, initially as a potential therapy for heart failure as well as HTN. His group at Ardian in Palo Alto, California, created a novel radiofrequency-based catheter ablation system. This interest, coupled with data from Esler and others,[2,3] suggests that biochemical changes in animal models of sympathetic denervation may be useful in HTN patients and led to the creation of a radiofrequency energy–based catheter. This catheter was designed as a 6-French guide and 0.014-in guide wire–compatible, single-point ablation catheter coupled to a generator, to be deployed in the renal arteries (Fig. 1). This system underwent extensive animal testing and eventually human use by the mid-2000s.

Early animal work was promising: in a swine HTN model, renal tissue norepinephrine levels were markedly reduced after denervation. In addition, vascular endothelial damage was transient within the renal arteries at the sites of ablation as shown by pathologic review, and there was no evidence of stenosis or luminal encroachment. Initial work in humans began in Australia by Krum and colleagues[4] demonstrated the safety of RDN as well as providing a glimpse at the biochemical changes after denervation. Their work, as well as others', suggested that measurements of norepinephrine spillover within the kidney or measured in the whole body could

Stanford University Interventional Cardiology, Room H-2103, 300 Pasteur Drive, Stanford, CA 94305, USA
E-mail address: dplee@stanford.edu

Intervent Cardiol Clin 9 (2020) 483–488
https://doi.org/10.1016/j.iccl.2020.07.004
2211-7458/20/© 2020 Elsevier Inc. All rights reserved.

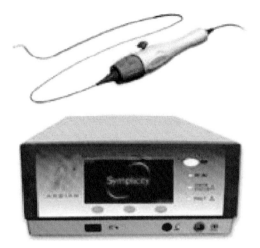

Fig. 1. Original SYMPLICITY (Flex) catheter system (Ardian). (*Courtesy of* Ardian, Mountain View, CA; with permission.)

demonstrate a reduction in sympathetic overactivity often seen in patients with HTN,[3] laying the groundwork for further studies in treating HTN. No detrimental effect on plasma renin or renal blood flow was demonstrated. In addition, the safety of bilateral RDN, as opposed to staged unilateral RDN, was shown in early feasibility.

CLINICAL TRIALS

As a result, the first formal clinical trial of RDN was the SYMPLICITY HTN-1 study.[5,6] In this study, 150 patients with resistant HTN were treated in an open-label fashion with RDN using the Ardian catheter. There was a clear and demonstrable reduction in office blood pressure (BP), which was durable out to 3-year follow-up. Initial reduction within the first 6 months was 22/10 mm Hg from a baseline, extending to 31/16 mm Hg at 36 months, suggesting a gradual reduction in BP, which lasts over an extended period of time. Much enthusiasm greeted this first report and a second trial, SYMPLICITY HTN-2,[7] was initiated to further gather proof that RDN could be a potential commercial therapy for HTN. In this randomized, crossover design trial, patients were selected to receive RDN initially or at 6 months after entering the trial. The results in both groups showed that RDN reduced office BP by (32/12 mm Hg in the initial treated group and 24/8 mm Hg in the crossover) at 6 months, with a gradual further reduction in BP at 30 months, as had been noted in the SYMPLICITY HTN-1 trial. In addition, the overall response rate to RDN was noted to be approximately 75% when defined

as a reduction of 10 mm Hg from baseline (63% when defined as a −20 mm Hg threshold) at 6 months.

As a result of these promising findings, a pivotal clinical trial, SYMPLICITY HTN-3,[8] was approved by the US Food and Drug Administration; 90 sites from across the United States were selected and a total of 530 patients were included in the trial. The design differed from the prior SYMPLICITY studies with the important addition of a sham control group (with crossover) in a 2:1 randomization scheme. In addition to office BP, 24-hour ambulatory BP also was measured. Patient selection was guided by office BP between 150 mm Hg and 180 mm Hg systolic despite multiple medications and age between 18 years and 80 years of age. Patients were screened to rule out secondary causes of HTN. The proceduralists were a mix of experienced and inexperienced operators but all were proctored during the cases. Patients also were managed in a double-blind fashion, with the catheterization laboratory operator handing off postprocedural follow-up to an experienced HTN specialist. The primary endpoint was the difference in office systolic BP at 6 months compared with baseline.

The results of this landmark trial were disappointing. In the end, the final results showed a decrease in office BP in the treatment group (n = 353) from a baseline of 179.7 mm Hg systolic to 165.6 mm Hg at 6 months (−14.2 mm Hg). The sham control group had a baseline of 180 mm Hg, which decreased to 168.4 mm Hg at 6-month follow-up (−11.6 mm Hg), leading to a net −2.39 mm Hg difference between the 2 groups (P = .255). In addition, the 24-hour ambulatory BPs also were not significantly different. Safety was positive, with only 2 events in both groups. Subsequent analysis of the RDN treatment group's failure to achieve significant difference in office BP focused on (1) completeness of the denervation, that is, achieving a quadrantic ablation circumferentially around the renal artery[9]; (2) relatively poor drug adherence in both groups, more specifically the use of spironolactone in the control group; and (3) the inclusion of isolated systolic HTN patients,[10] which may have been a confounder. The mean number of ablations per patient was 14. The disappointment of the result dissuaded several companies from further developing RDN technology. Medtronic (Santa Rosa, California), which had acquired Ardian, was left to re-evaluate their program and its future.

Despite the negative results, the new field of RDN was spurring new interest in understanding the basic mechanism(s) of action and furthering anatomic study as well. The initial technique of highlighting and treating the body of the main renal artery in retrospect may have been inadequate, with studies suggesting that the sympathetic nerves surrounding the renal arteries generally are up to 7 mm to 8 mm from the vessel wall. In addition, the concept of a nerve plexus, previously thought arise most often near the renal artery ostium along the aortic border, was much less common than had been believed. These data and the observation that distal renal artery and branch ablation perhaps yielded a better result because of the closer proximity of the renal sympathetic nerves while moving out toward the renal cortex persuaded a change in the technique to achieve more complete ablation.[11,12] The observation that patients with combined systolic and diastolic HTN responded better to RDN was noted.[13] In addition, an improved catheter, the Spyral catheter (https://global.medtronic.com/xg-en/healthcare-professionals/products/cardiovascular/renal-denervation/symplicity.html) was developed by Medtronic to better deliver quadrantic ablation with 4 radiofrequency elements in a spiral design; it remains 6-French and 0.014-in guide wire compatible. In addition to Medtronic, other companies, notably Recor Medical (Palo Alto, CA) and Ablative Solutions (Kalamazoo, MI), continued to develop competing technologies within the field.

RECENT TRIALS

With a set of catheter enhancements as well as more rigorous trial design, the SPYRAL studies were launched. These protocols focused the effort on hypertensive patients with 3 or fewer medications and excluded patients with isolated systolic HTN. In addition, patients with resistant HTN, who had been the target of the SYMPLICITY trials, also were now excluded. Two studies, SYPRAL HTN-OFF and SPYRAL HTN-ON,[14] were designed to study patients either taking no medications (OFF) or those with 1 to 3 medications (ON) and BP measurements in the 150-180/>=90 mm Hg. To address the role of compliance, urinary screening for antihypertensive drugs was mandated within the trial protocol. Protocol-defined use of antihypertensive medications also was enforced more rigorously and patients taking spironolactone were excluded. Guideline-directed medical therapy, including lifestyle changes, also were encouraged. Enrollment in these studies, although relatively robust, reflected a large screening effort to find patients suitable for the studies, with enrollment rates of approximately only 10% to 20% of the total screening population. The use of the new catheter beyond the main renal artery was now expanded to branch vessels as well. Finally, a limited number of sites (44) from around the world were included in the SPYRAL protocols to ensure experienced RDN operators.

The initial report of the SPYRAL studies was derived from the first 80 randomized patients in the SPYRAL HTN-OFF pilot protocol.[15] The 3-month BP outcomes were measured in the 38 treated and 42 sham control patients. In the patients who underwent RDN, the office BP was noted to decrease by an average of 10.0/5.3 mm Hg with a 24-hour ambulatory reduction from baseline by 5.5/4.8 mm Hg. The sham control group fell 2.3/0.3 mm Hg in office BP (systolic difference vs RDN treated 7.7 mm Hg; $P = .02$) and 0.5/0.4 in the 24-hour ambulatory BP (systolic vs RDN; $P = .04$). A similar report from the initial 80 randomized patients in SPYRAL HTN-ON pilot[16] yielded a similar positive comparison of RDN versus sham control patients with a reduction of 6.8 mm Hg systolic office BP ($P = .02$). With the targeting the main renal artery as well as its branches, the total numbers of ablations per patient in both trials were 43.8 in OFF and 45.9 in ON, a marked increase from SYMPLICITY HTN-3. These 2 pilot studies have spurred the SPYRAL protocols to become pivotal trials. The SPYRAL HTN-OFF MED Pivotal trial[17] recently was reported, enrolling a total of 353 patients at 44 sites, including the original 80 patients from the pilot trial; 166 patients underwent RDN with 165 in the sham control group. The mean number of ablations per patient was 46.9. The primary endpoint of 24-hour ambulatory BP office systolic BP at 3 months showed a 4.7/3/7 mm Hg BP drop in the RDN group versus a 0.6/0.8 mm Hg drop in the control group, a difference of 4.0/3.1 between the 2 groups ($P<.001$). The office BP were similarly impressive (6.6/4.4 mm Hg difference between RDN and sham; $P<.001$). With respect to safety, 1 patient in the RDN group was hospitalized for hypertensive crisis and 1 patient in the control arm suffered a stroke within the first 3 months after randomization. There were no vascular complications. Other interesting findings included protocol-mandated medication adjustments in 9.6% of the RDN patients and 17.0% in the control group ($P = .049$). Compliance with being off all antihypertensive medications was 91.2% in the RDN group and 94.9% in the control. The SPYRAL HTN-ON MED Pivotal trial remains in enrollment at this time.

In addition to the SPYRAL trials, catheter-based ultrasound denervation has emerged with the RADIANCE trials. The Paradise catheter (ReCor Medical; https://www.recormedical.com/our-technology) utilizes a 7-French, 0.014-in guide wire compatible design with 3 ultrasound elements to disperse heat energy across the vessel wall into the renal adventitia to denervate the renal sympathetic nerves. One unique property of this catheter system is that it is radial vascular access compliant. The RADIANCE-HTN SOLO 2-month results[18] were reported within a limited pilot study, randomizing 146 patients with moderate systolic and diastolic HTN (140–180/90–110 mm Hg) on 2 or fewer medications to RDN (n = 74) or sham (n = 72). The primary endpoint was daytime ambulatory BP and this was reduced in the treatment arm by 5.1 mm Hg versus 2.6 mm Hg in the control group (difference 2.5 mm Hg; $P = .01$); 24-hour ambulatory BP differed by 4.1 mm Hg ($P<.001$), also favoring the treatment group. The 6-month results[19] were consistent with these results. This trial since has expanded to a pivotal trial (RADIANCE II). The RADIANCE-HTN TRIO trial, which includes patients taking 3 or more antihypertensive medications, is studying the role of ultrasound-based denervation and recently has completed enrollment.

Another catheter-based approach is being developed by Ablative Solutions (Kalamazoo, Michigan; https://ablativesolutions.com/index.php/us/physicians/peregrine-system-infusion-catheter). Their Peregrine system utilizes a set of 3 microneedles, which, after appropriate positioning in the main renal artery, are deployed through the vessel wall. Desiccated ethanol, a direct nerve toxin, then is injected into the renal adventitia to perform the denervation. Data from the open-label, European multicenter Peregrine Post-Market Study showed an 11.0–mm Hg reduction in 24-hour ambulatory and 18–mm Hg reduction in office BP 6 months after treatment in a small number of nonrandomized patients (n = 45).[20] TARGET-BP I is a worldwide, multicenter pivotal study, which is now under way, randomizing patients with moderate HTN taking 2 to 5 medications, with TARGET BP OFF-MED studying European patients who are not taking medication for HTN. Both of these studies include blinding and sham control.

DISCUSSION

RDN has had a progressive if interesting course as it approaches commercial approval. The challenge of defining the right study population has been difficult, but with perseverance a clearer picture has emerged. Patients with moderate HTN on 3 or fewer medicines are likely to be the first to have the opportunity to undergo RDN commercially in the United States. With the failure of SYMPLICITY HTN-3, interest in RDN had waned but the combination of new technology as well as a refinement of the study population and protocols has led to success within the SPYRAL trials and promise for the RADIANCE and TARGET trials. Safety across all the studies appears to be excellent. There still are many questions, however, to be answered.

As discussed previously, not all patients in the studies are responding as expected to treatment; success rates generally are in the 70% to 80% range. This rebirth of RDN also has spurred further interest in understanding the differences between responders and nonresponders: several small trials currently are investigating this from multiple perspectives, including genetic testing, proteomics, nerve mapping, and other modalities. In addition, expectations need to be managed: for instance, for patients taking medication, should they expect to have their medications reduced and by how much or many? For patients who are off their prior medications, how durable is the procedure and should they expect to avoid medications for the rests of their life? These are common questions for patients enrolling in these studies.

As more data are accumulated, questions regarding the relative efficacy between the different treatment modalities of radiofrequency, ultrasound, and alcohol ablation are likely to arise. At this point, it is unclear whether any of these catheter-based treatment strategies is superior compared with the other modalities. The reduction in BP across all of the trials appears to be similar, suggesting the most important parameter for success is the ablation itself as opposed to the mode of treatment. There are some differences in terms of catheter size requirements and lengths of procedure, and these may in the end become more of a differentiator in determining the choice of modality rather than efficacy.

It should be expected that not all interested patients will be candidates for RDN. The large amount of screening to yield a relatively small percentage of study-eligible patients has been a barrier for the trials, and moving outside the expected indications may be detrimental for RDN commercial success. A team-based approach with HTN specialists and interventionalists working in conjunction with primary care providers is the current best strategy for patient recruitment and this likely will continue with commercial approval.

There also are other approaches to RDN, including other catheter systems as well as endoscopic approaches, which currently are in development. All appear to be feasible and have begun clinical trials outside the United States and Europe. They also may yield important new information as they mature.

Finally, although the focus of RDN has been on HTN, there are other potential clinical areas of interest that may benefit from RDN: these include atrial fibrillation (during atrial fibrillation ablation),[21] heart failure,[22] and diabetes.[23] As RDN gains a foothold in HTN, these other clinical maladies likely will be studied as well.

SUMMARY

RDN is still relatively young but has been an important and exciting new therapy for HTN. The initial excitement and fervor with the early trials markedly waned after SYMPLICITY HTN-3. A refocus on the problems within that trial led to improvements in technique, technology, and patient selection. As the newer trials have shown success, there is a renewed and palpable interest in RDN. There still are many questions to be answered but the future appears bright, and patients and physicians should look forward to this new and safe procedure for treating HTN.

DISCLOSURE

Medtronic (research grant and consultant) and Ablative Solutions (research grant).

REFERENCES

1. Smithwick RH, Thompson JE. Splanchicectomy for essential hypertension: results in 1266 cases. JAMA 1953;152:1501–4.
2. Esler M. The sympathetic system and hypertension. Am J Hypertens 2000;13:S4, 99S–105S.
3. Schlaich MP, Lambert E, Kaye DM, et al. Sympathetic augmentation in hypertension: role of nerve firing, norepinephrine reuptake, and angiotensin neuromodulation. Hypertension 2004;43:169–75.
4. Krum H, Schlaich M, Whitbourn R, et al. Catheter-based renal sympathetic denervation for resistant hypertension: a multicentre safety and proof-of-principle cohort study. Lancet 2009;373:1275–81.
5. Schlaich MP, Sobotka PA, Krum H, et al. Renal sympathetic-nerve ablation for uncontrolled hypertension. N Engl J Med 2009;36(9):932–4.
6. Symplicity HTN-1 Investigators. Catheter-based renal sympathetic denervation for resistant hypertension: durability of blood pressure reduction out to 24 months. Hypertension 2011;57:911–7.
7. Esler MD, Krum H, Schlaich M, et al, for the Symplicity HTN-2 Investigators. Renal sympathetic denervation for treatment of drug-resistant hypertension: one-year results from the Symplicity HTN-2 randomized, controlled trial. Circulation 2012;126:2976–82.
8. Bhatt DL, Kandzari DE, O'Neill WW, et al, for the Symplicity HTN-3 investigators. A controlled trial of renal denervation for resistant hypertension. N Engl J Med 2014;370:1393–401.
9. Mahfoud F, Tunev S, Ewen S, et al. Impact of lesion placement on efficacy and safety of catheter-based radiofrequency renal denervation. J Am Coll Cardiol 2015;66:1766–75.
10. Mahfoud F, Bakris G, Bhatt DL, et al. Reduced blood pressure-lowering effect of catheter-based renal denervation in patients with isolated systolic hypertension: data from SYMPLICITY HTN-3 and the global SYMPLICITY Registry. Eur Heart J 2017;38(2):93–100.
11. Petrov I. "Y-pattern, 4-quadrant, multiple points" is the answer. Cardiovasc Revasc Med 2018. https://doi.org/10.1016/j.carrev.2018.12.005.
12. Fengler K, Ewen S, Höllriegel R, et al. Blood pressure response to main renal artery and combined main renal artery plus branch renal denervation in patients with resistant hypertension. J Am Heart Assoc 2017;6:e006196.
13. Ewen S, Ukena C, Linz D, et al. Reduced effect of percutaneous renal denervation on blood pressure in patients with isolated systolic hypertension. Hypertension 2015;65:193–9.
14. Kandzari D, Kario K, Mahfoud F, et al. The SPYRAL HTN global clinical trial program: rationale and design for studies of renal denervation in the absence (SPYRAL HTN OFF-MED) and presence (SPYRAL HTN ON-MED) of antihypertensive medications. Am Heart J 2016;171:82–91.
15. Townsend RR, Mahfoud F, Kandzari DE, et al, for the SPYRAL HTN-OFF MED Investigators. Catheter-based renal denervation in patients with uncontrolled hypertension in the absence of antihypertensive medications (SPYRAL HTN-OFF MED): a randomised, sham-controlled, proof-of-concept trial. Lancet 2017;390:2160–70.
16. Kandzari DE, Böhm M, Mahfoud F, et al, for the SPYRAL HTN-ON MED Investigators. Effect of renal denervation on blood pressure in the presence of antihypertensive drugs: 6-month efficacy and safety results from the SPYRAL HTN-ON MED proof-of-concept randomised trial. Lancet 2018;391:2346–55.
17. Böhm M, Kario K, Kandzari DE, et al, for the SPYRAL HTN-OFF MED Investigators. Efficacy of catheter-based renal denervation in the absence

of antihypertensive medications (SPYRAL HTN-OFF MED Pivotal): a multicentre, randomised, sham-controlled trial. Lancet 2020;395:1444–51.

18. Azizi M, Schmieder RE, Mahfoud F, et al. Endovascular ultrasound renal denervation to treat hypertension (RADIANCE-HTN SOLO): a multicentre, international, single-blind, randomised, sham-controlled trial. Lancet 2018;391:2335–45.

19. Azizi M, Schmieder RE, Mahfoud F, et al. Six-month results of treatment-blinded medication titration for hypertension control following randomization to endovascular ultrasound renal denervation or a sham procedure in the RADIANCE-HTN SOLO trial. Circulation 2019;139:2542–53.

20. Mahfoud F, Renkin J, Sievert H, et al. Alcohol-mediated renal denervation using the Peregrine system infusion catheter for treatment of hypertension. JACC Cardiovasc Interv 2020;13:471–84.

21. Steinberg JS, Shabanov V, Ponomarev D, et al. Effect of renal denervation and catheter ablation vs catheter ablation alone on atrial fibrillation recurrence among patients with paroxysmal atrial fibrillation and hypertension: the ERADICATE-AF randomized clinical trial. JAMA 2020;323:248–55.

22. Fukuta H, Goto T, Wakami K, et al. Effects of catheter-based renal denervation on heart failure with reduced ejection fraction: a systematic review and meta-analysis. Heart Fail Rev 2017;22:657–64.

23. Mahfoud F, Ewen S, Ukena C, et al. Expanding the indication spectrum: renal denervation in diabetes. Eurointervention 2013;9(Suppl R):R117–21.

The Role of Aspirin After High-Risk Percutaneous Coronary Intervention

The Ticagrelor with Aspirin or Alone in High-Risk Patients After Coronary Intervention Clinical Trial Experience

Zain Ul Abideen Asad, MD, Usman Baber, MD, MS*

KEYWORDS

- Aspirin • P2Y$_{12}$ inhibitors • Percutaneous coronary intervention • Acute coronary syndrome
- Stable ischemic heart disease

KEY POINTS

- Historical studies that included aspirin as a background therapy after percutaneous coronary intervention (PCI) introduced the current paradigm of dual antiplatelet therapy (DAPT).
- The clinical basis for aspirin-free strategies is predicated on lowering bleeding without compromising anti-ischemic efficacy with P2Y$_{12}$ inhibitor therapy alone.
- In cohorts of patients not at high bleeding risk, several clinical trials have shown superior clinical outcomes with P2Y$_{12}$ inhibitor monotherapy after a short duration of DAPT as compared with continuation of DAPT.
- Subgroup analyses of these trials suggest P2Y$_{12}$ inhibitor monotherapy with Ticagrelor may improve safety without compromising the efficacy in high ischemic risk patients with diabetes, acute coronary syndrome and those undergoing complex PCI.
- Decisions with respect to antithrombotic therapy should be tailored according to clinical phenotype and/or genotype.

INTRODUCTION

Percutaneous coronary intervention (PCI) is the most commonly performed invasive cardiac procedure for patients with ischemic heart disease.[1,2] Since the original description of coronary angioplasty by Andreas Gruntzig in 1978, this procedure has evolved considerably in terms of technique, equipment, and adjunctive pharmacotherapy.[3,4] Over the past half century, aspirin has been an integral part of primary and secondary prevention of cardiovascular (CV) disease.

Aspirin has a well-established role in the secondary prevention of adverse cardiac events in patients with ischemic heart disease.[5,6] For patients undergoing PCI, American College of Cardiology/American Heart Association (ACC/AHA) guidelines recommended dual antiplatelet therapy (DAPT) for secondary prevention of adverse CV events, for at least 6 months in stable ischemic heart disease (SIHD) and 12 months for acute coronary syndrome (ACS).[5–9] For patients with low risk of bleeding and higher ischemic risk, longer duration of DAPT consisting of aspirin and a P2Y$_{12}$ inhibitor can be

Cardiovascular Disease Section, Department of Medicine, University of Oklahoma Health Sciences Center, Andrews Academic Tower, Suite 5400, 800 Stanton L. Young Boulevard, Oklahoma City, OK 73104, USA
* Corresponding author.
E-mail address: Usman-baber@ouhsc.edu

2211-7458/20/© 2020 Elsevier Inc. All rights reserved.

considered.[10] For patients at a higher risk of bleeding, DAPT maybe discontinued after 3 months in SIHD and after 6 months in ACS.

However, aspirin use is associated with bleeding complications and therefore newer antithrombotic regimens have been tested that may increase the overall benefit to the patient by reducing the bleeding risk and offering better or similar efficacy. These new regimens include addition of P2Y$_{12}$ inhibitors and oral anticoagulants in various combinations and durations to a background of aspirin or an aspirin-free strategy. Since the last major update to clinical practice guidelines for patients with SIHD and ACS, multiple large trials testing different durations of DAPT followed by aspirin monotherapy, P2Y$_{12}$ monotherapy, and their combinations with oral anticoagulants (dual therapy vs triple therapy) have been conducted. This emerging evidence has raised important questions about the role of aspirin in patients undergoing PCI. Patient-specific ischemic and bleeding risk factors and concomitant use of anticoagulants make decisions regarding aspirin use in patients undergoing PCI very complex. In this article, we discuss the role of aspirin in the secondary prevention of CV events for patients undergoing PCI in light of recent clinical trials and provide a simplified approach that allows clinicians to tailor this recent evidence to individual patients.

HISTORICAL PERSPECTIVE

Pooled analyses of randomized studies among patients with established atherosclerotic vascular disease (ASCVD) have shown that aspirin significantly reduces recurrent vascular events as compared with placebo or active control.[11] As a consequence, pivotal trials evaluating different antithrombotic regiments in the early PCI era mandated the use of aspirin as a foundational antiplatelet drug to which additional agents were then added.[12] Results from these studies found that the addition of a P2Y$_{12}$ inhibitor to aspirin (ie, DAPT), was the most efficacious strategy for lowering recurrent thrombosis following PCI as compared with aspirin alone or aspirin coupled with an oral anticoagulant. However, the benefits with respect to ischemic events attributed to DAPT in prior studies reflect the incremental efficacy of P2Y$_{12}$ inhibition, not aspirin.[13] This distinction is clinically meaningful, as aspirin increases bleeding risk and hemorrhagic complications after PCI are associated with a significant and durable risk for mortality.[14] Beyond the clinical impact of bleeding, safer stent platforms and adjunctive

pharmacotherapy have fundamentally altered the risk benefit calculus for prolonged exposure to DAPT after PCI. In this regard, numerous clinical trials have evaluated novel therapeutic strategies, including P2Y$_{12}$ inhibitor monotherapy, in an effort to mitigate aspirin-related bleeding while not compromising efficacy from potent platelet inhibition.[15–18]

P2Y$_{12}$ INHIBITOR MONOTHERAPY AFTER PERCUTANEOUS CORONARY INTERVENTION: RANDOMIZED EVIDENCE

To date, at least 5 randomized clinical trials have examined the safety and efficacy of P2Y$_{12}$ inhibitor monotherapy after a short duration of DAPT following PCI (Table 1). Two studies included East Asian patients and maintained P2Y$_{12}$ inhibition with clopidogrel alone after 1 or 3 months of DAPT. In both trials, bleeding was reduced over 1 year with clopidogrel monotherapy as compared with continued DAPT without an apparent increase in ischemic events. However, the modest sample sizes and concerns regarding pharmacodynamic variability with clopidogrel precludes robust conclusions regarding the safety of this strategy after PCI. In the GLOBAL LEADERS trial, 15,968 patients treated with Biolimus A9 drug-eluting stent (DES) were randomized to a conventional antiplatelet strategy versus ticagrelor monotherapy after 1 month of DAPT.[17] Over 23 months, the primary endpoint of death or Q-wave myocardial infarction (MI) was not significantly reduced with the experimental strategy (3.81% vs 4.37%, rate ratio 0.87, P = .073). Somewhat counterintuitively, there were also no reductions in site-reported bleeding between treatment arms.

In contrast to these studies, TWILIGHT (Ticagrelor With Aspirin or Alone in High-Risk Patients After Coronary Intervention) was a randomized, double-blind placebo-controlled trial that enrolled high-risk patients undergoing PCI with DES from disparate global regions (North America, Europe, Asia).[15] Trial enrollment required the presence of at least 1 clinical and 1 angiographic high-risk criterion (Table 2). These features were prespecified and protocol-defined to generate a trial cohort with sufficient risk to reliably detect differences between allocated treatments. In addition, all adverse events were adjudicated in a blinded fashion by an independent committee. Following successful PCI with DES, enrolled patients received 3 months of open-label DAPT with ticagrelor plus aspirin. Adherent and event-free patients were then randomized in a double-blind fashion to aspirin or

Table 1
Trials evaluating 1 month to 3 months' duration of dual antiplatelet therapy followed by aspirin or P2Y$_{12}$ monotherapy

Duration & Strategy	1 Month DAPT	P2Y12 Monotherapy After 1 Month of DAPT		P2Y12 Monotherapy After 3 Months of DAPT		
Study	ONYX ONE[40]	GLOBAL LEADERS[17]	STOP DAPT-2[18]	SMART CHOICE[16]	TWILIGHT[15]	TICO[41]
Intervention arm	Resolute ONYX DES	1 mo DAPT then 23 mo Ticagrelor only	1 mo DAPT then P2Y$_{12}$ monotherapy	3 mo DAPT then P2Y$_{12}$ only for 12 mo	3 mo DAPT then Ticagrelor only for 12 mo	3 mo DAPT then Ticagrelor only for 12 mo
Control arm	Bio Freedom DCS	12 mo DAPT	12 mo DAPT	12 mo DAPT	12 mo DAPT	12 mo DAPT
Sample size	1996	7980/7988	1500/1509	1495/1498	3555/3564	1527/1529
Age	74	64.5/64.6	68.1/69.1	64.6/64.4	65.2/65.1	61
ACS (%)	51%	47/46.8	37.7/38.6	58.2/58.2	63.9/65.7	100/100 (STEMI 36%)
Prior PCI (%)		32.7/32.7	33.5/35.1		42.3/42	135/127
MVD (%)		25.7/24.9	39/38	50.1/49.0	63.9/61.6	9/8
Diabetes (%)				38.2/36.8	37.1/36.5	27
Follow-up	1 y	2 y	1 y	1 y	1 y	1 y
Primary Outcome	CV death, MI, ST	Death or Q-wave MI	CV death, MI, definite ST, stroke, TIMI major or minor bleeding	Death, MI, Stroke	BARC 2, 3,5 bleeding	Death, MI, ST, Stroke, TVR, TIMI Major bleeding
Conclusion	CV death, MI, ST for Resolute vs Bio Freedom was 17.1% vs 16.9% (noninferior 0.011)	Not superior in preventing all-cause mortality or new Q-wave MI at 2 y	Superior for reducing CV and bleeding events	Noninferior in preventing MACE	Lower incidence of bleeding without increasing risk of MI, stroke, death	Superior

Abbreviations: ACS, acute coronary syndrome; BARC, bleeding academic research consortium; CV, cardiovascular; DAPT, dual antiplatelet therapy; DCS, drug-coated stent; MACE, major adverse cardiac events; MI, myocardial infarction; MVD, multi vessel disease; PCI, percutaneous coronary intervention; STEMI, ST-elevation myocardial infarction; TIMI, thrombolysis in myocardial infarction; TVR, target vessel revascularization.

Table 2	
TWILIGHT trial inclusion criteria	
Clinical Inclusion Criteria	**Angiographic Inclusion Criteria**
Age $\geq$65 y	Multivessel coronary artery disease
Recent (>3 d) presentation with acute coronary syndrome with clinical stabilization and decreasing cardiac enzymes	Target lesion requiring total stent length >30 mm
Established vascular disease defined as previous myocardial infarction, documented peripheral arterial disease or revascularization for coronary artery disease/peripheral arterial disease	Bifurcation lesions with Medina X, X, 1 classification requiring at least 2 stents
Diabetes mellitus treated with medications or insulin	SYNTAX score $\geq$23
Chronic kidney disease defined as an estimated glomerular filtration rate <60 mL/min per 1.73 m^2 or creatinine clearance (CrCl) <60 mL/min	Left main ($\geq$50%) or proximal left anterior descending artery (70%) lesion
	Calcified target lesions requiring atherectomy
Patients were required to meet at least 1 clinical criterion and 1 angiographic criterion for inclusion.	

matching placebo with continuation of ticagrelor for an additional year. Ticagrelor monotherapy significantly reduced clinically relevant bleeding academic research consortium (BARC) type 2, 3, or 5 bleeding by 44% (4% vs 7.1%; $P<.001$). More severe BARC type 3 or 5 bleeding was reduced by a similar magnitude (1% vs 2%; hazard ratio [HR] 0.49). Moreover, noninferiority was maintained for the key secondary endpoint of all-cause death, MI, or stroke (3.9% vs 3.9%; $P_{NI} <0.001$). Results for both bleeding and ischemic endpoints were consistent across different clinical subgroups and enrolling region. The sample size, design features, and uniform results of TWILIGHT provide the most robust randomized evidence to date supporting the use of $P2Y_{12}$ inhibitor monotherapy following a short duration of DAPT in select patients undergoing PCI.

HIGH-RISK PATIENTS

The construct of high risk in the setting of PCI involves clinical (acute vs stable), procedural (stent length), and anatomic (coronary calcification) domains. Several studies have shown that prolonged durations of DAPT in such patients lowers residual thrombotic risk, albeit with excess bleeding.[19,20] The utility of bleeding-avoidance strategies in such patients may be inferred from several studies and subgroup analyses of randomized trials. Among patients with

ST-elevation myocardial infarction (STEMI), a short duration of DAPT followed by aspirin monotherapy was associated with an excess risk of recurrent MI as compared with continued DAPT.[21] In contrast, early withdrawal of aspirin followed by ticagrelor monotherapy has emerged as a safer alternative to DAPT in patients with ACS.

Acute Coronary Syndrome

Subgroup analyses from both GLOBAL LEADERS and TWILIGHT have shown consistent results with ticagrelor monotherapy among patients with ACS enrolled in each respective study (Fig. 1). Among 7487 ACS patients enrolled in GLOBAL LEADERS, ticagrelor alone reduced BARC type 3 or 5 bleeding by 48% (0.8% vs 1.5%; $P = .004$). TWILIGHT enrolled 4614 patients with non–ST-elevation ACS (unstable angina or non-STEMI). The bleeding-related benefit of ticagrelor monotherapy was accentuated in these patients ($P_{int} = .03$) whereas the rates of ischemic events were not different between groups (4.3% vs 4.4%; $P = .84$).[22] Results were consistent even among patients with non–ST-elevation ACS with multiple high-risk features in whom the 1-year ischemic event rates were substantial. The results of the TICO (Ticagrelor Monotherapy After 3 Months in the Patients Treated With New Generation Sirolimus Stent for Acute Coronary Syndrome) trial were consistent with these findings from TWILIGHT

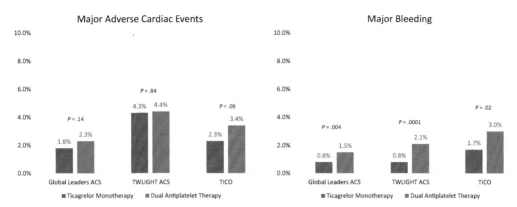

Fig. 1. Outcomes in patients with acute coronary syndrome in Ticagrelor monotherapy trials. For GLOBAL LEADERS ACS post-hoc analysis, the major adverse cardiac events included death, new-Q-wave myocardial infarction or stroke and major bleeding included BARC 3 or 5 bleeding. For TWILIGHT-ACS the major adverse cardiac events included death, myocardial infarction or stroke and major bleeding included BARC 3 or 5 bleeding. For TICO the major adverse cardiac events included death, myocardial infarction, stent thrombosis, stroke or target vessel revascularization and major bleeding included TIMI major bleeding.

subgroup analysis. TICO was designed to examine the effect of ticagrelor monotherapy after 3 months of DAPT in patients with ACS exclusively. The trial enrolled 3056 patients (36% with STEMI) treated with an ultrathin bioresorbable-polymer DES. Over 1 year, the composite net adverse clinical outcome (death, MI, stent thrombosis, stroke, target vessel revascularization, TIMI [Thrombolysis in Myocardial Infarction] major bleeding) was significantly reduced with ticagrelor monotherapy (3.9% vs 5.9%; $P = .01$). Importantly, rates of stent thrombosis were low and did not vary between groups (0.4% vs 0.3%; $P = .53$). In aggregate, these results challenge the conventional paradigm mandating the use of long-term aspirin in all patients as a component of DAPT following PCI.

Diabetes Mellitus
The presence of diabetes mellitus increases thrombotic risk after PCI, even among patients treated with newer-generation DES. Risk is particularly accentuated among patients with insulin-treated diabetes.[23,24] Comorbid conditions that enhance bleeding risk, such as older age and renal impairment, are also prevalent among diabetic individuals, complicating therapeutic decision-making with respect to DAPT. In this regard, a bleeding-avoidance strategy that preserves the benefits of intensive $P2Y_{12}$ inhibition while lowering aspirin-related bleeding may offer unique advantages. This hypothesis was examined in a prespecified analysis of the 2620 diabetic patients enrolled in the TWILIGHT trial. Approximately 27% of the cohort was treated with insulin and comorbid conditions that increase risk for either bleeding or

thrombosis, such as chronic kidney disease ($\sim$21%) and multivessel coronary artery disease ($\sim$68%), were highly prevalent. Ticagrelor monotherapy reduced the risk of clinically relevant bleeding by 35% without increasing ischemic events as compared with ticagrelor plus aspirin (4.6% vs 5.9%; $P = .14$). Individual ischemic endpoints, including all-cause death (1.3% vs 2.0%), MI (3.1% vs 4.1%), and stent thrombosis (0.5% vs 0.7%), were not increased among those randomized to placebo, supporting the safety of ticagrelor monotherapy in such patients.[25] Hence, these findings provide randomized evidence supporting a short duration of DAPT followed by ticagrelor monotherapy in complex patients with diabetes mellitus undergoing PCI.

Complex Percutaneous Coronary Intervention
Several studies have shown the prognostic impact of either procedural or lesion-based parameters following PCI.[19,26] In a post hoc analysis of the TWILIGHT trial, Dangas and colleagues[27] examined the effect of ticagrelor monotherapy among patients undergoing complex PCI, defined as PCI with at least 1 of the following features: 3 vessels treated; $\geq$3 lesions treated; total stent length greater than 60 mm; bifurcation lesion with 2 stents implanted; use of any atherectomy device; left main target vessel; venous or arterial bypass graft target vessel; or chronic total occlusion target lesion. These criteria were derived and modified from a similar set of validated parameters.[28] Approximately 33% of TWILIGHT participants were characterized as receiving complex PCI based

on this definition. Patients undergoing complex PCI were older with a higher prevalence of renal impairment, anemia, and prior coronary revascularization as compared with their counterparts undergoing noncomplex PCI. Consistent with other subgroup analyses, ticagrelor monotherapy significantly reduced the rate of clinically relevant bleeding (4.2% vs 7.7%; $P<.001$). Perhaps more importantly, though, rates of all-cause death, MI, or stroke were numerically, albeit not significantly, reduced with ticagrelor monotherapy (3.8% vs 4.9%; 95% confidence interval 0.52–1.15). A nonsignificant trend toward lower stent thrombosis was also observed with ticagrelor alone (0.4% vs 0.8%). One unexpected result from this analysis was that the overall rate of death, MI, or stroke was not substantially higher than that observed in the overall trial cohort. This finding may reflect the importance of procedural parameters in influencing early versus later ischemic events after PCI.[29] As patients were randomized after 3 months in TWILIGHT, it is plausible that the adverse effect of complex procedures was somewhat attenuated.

EXPERIMENTAL EVIDENCE

Experimental studies provide a physiologic basis and biological rationale for the lack of incremental thrombosis associated with aspirin withdrawal while maintaining ticagrelor alone. Pharmacodynamic investigations have shown that aspirin provides limited additional platelet inhibition in platelets isolated from healthy volunteers treated with potent $P2Y_{12}$ inhibitors. Other experimental studies conducted in animals using a variety of thrombogenic stimuli suggest a limited effect of aspirin in reducing thrombus formation on a background of ongoing $P2Y_{12}$ blockade.[30] These results are concordant with those of a nested substudy within the TWILIGHT trial wherein ex vivo thrombus formation was examined under conditions of shear stress and dynamic flow, thereby overcoming limitations of earlier studies. In this report, 51 TWILIGHT study participants underwent ex vivo perfusion assays to measure thrombus area at a single center at the time of randomization when patients were on maintenance DAPT.[31] Approximately 1.5 months thereafter repeat assays were performed when patients were receiving either placebo or aspirin. Thrombus area was comparable between groups, suggesting that aspirin withdrawal does not modulate ex vivo blood thrombogenicity among high-risk patients treated with ticagrelor. However, markers sensitive to cyclooxygenase (COX)-1 blockade were increased among patients randomized to placebo. These findings provide physiologic corroboration to the clinical findings of no incremental thrombosis on aspirin withdrawal observed in the overall trial. Similarly, Franchi and colleagues[32] found that validated indices of blood thrombogenicity did not significantly vary following aspirin withdrawal among patients receiving different antithrombotic agents.

THERAPEUTIC SELECTION

Identifying the optimal treatment for appropriately selected patients is a natural goal of any medical decision-making process. With respect to antiplatelet therapy, the convergence of data examining unique patient cohorts, specific stent platforms, and therapeutic permutations has rendered such decisions quite nuanced and complex. For example, the Academic Research Consortium has defined high bleeding risk (HBR) as those patients with an estimated annualized risk for BARC type 3 or 5 bleeding of at least 4%.[33] The LEADERS FREE trial was the first randomized trial focused exclusively on patients with HBR. In this study, a polymer-free drug-coated stent (DCS) was compared with a bare metal stent (BMS) among patients with HBR receiving 1 month of DAPT followed by aspirin alone. The patient population was characterized by a mean age of 75 years and a 1-year BARC type 3 or 5 bleeding rate of approximately 7%. The primary safety outcome of cardiac death, MI, or stent thrombosis was significantly lower with the polymer-free DCS as compared with BMS (9.4% vs 12.9%; $P<.001$). In a separate report, the ONYX ONE investigators evaluated a different DES platform in patients with HBR receiving 1 month of DAPT. Most patients were transitioned to aspirin alone after 1 month, whereas $P2Y_{12}$ inhibitor monotherapy occurred predominantly in patients receiving concomitant oral anticoagulation. Trial participants were characterized by a mean age of 74 years and the 1-year BARC type 3 or 5 bleeding rate was approximately 4.6%, exceeding the HBR-ARC threshold of 4%. In aggregate, these studies suggest that in "true" HBR, patients may be optimally treated with a very short duration of DAPT and newer-generation DES. It is somewhat intuitive that in such patients there is a clinical imperative to minimize both the duration and intensity of platelet inhibition as much as possible.

In contrast to these reports, TWILIGHT participants displayed a mean age of 65 years and the

1-year rate of BARC type 3 or 5 bleeding was only 1.8%, suggesting that TWILIGHT enrolled a non-HBR cohort. Other studies examining $P2Y_{12}$ inhibitor monotherapy have also enrolled predominantly non-HBR patients per the established threshold set forth by the Academic Research Consortium. Finally, other studies enrolling relatively low-risk patients undergoing noncomplex PCI have found that a short duration of DAPT followed by aspirin alone may be sufficient as compared with continuation of DAPT.[34,35]

In an effort to consolidate recent results from these clinical trials, we propose a clinical algorithm to facilitate decision-making with respect to antiplatelet therapy after PCI (Fig. 2). In this schema, the first step is to identify patients with HBR and treat such individuals with a very short duration of DAPT (ie, 1 month) followed by aspirin alone vis à vis the LEADERS FREE and ONYX ONE studies. For non-HBR patients, it is necessary to then consider ischemic risk. For patients at low ischemic risk (ie, noncomplex PCI, non-ACS, single-vessel CAD), a 3-month to 6-month duration of DAPT followed by aspirin alone may be reasonable and aligns with current guidelines. However, for those patients at intermediate to high thrombotic risk, such as those fulfilling TWILIGHT inclusion criteria or presenting with ACS, a short duration of DAPT followed by $P2Y_{12}$ inhibitor monotherapy has emerged as a viable treatment strategy.

FUTURE DIRECTIONS

Most studies examining different antiplatelet strategies in the setting of PCI have followed patients for a relatively short duration (ie, 1–3 years); hence, the optimal antithrombotic regimen for long-term secondary prevention remains an active area of clinical investigation with equipoise for a variety of different treatment options. Patients with multiterritorial ASCVD derive a clear benefit with the addition of a low-dose direct oral anticoagulant to aspirin based on several large randomized trials.[36,37] In contrast, among patients with a history of prior MI, prolonged DAPT with ticagrelor plus aspirin was superior to aspirin alone for prevention of recurrent ischemic events. Whether or not $P2Y_{12}$ inhibitor monotherapy would yield a similar benefit without incurring excess bleeding risk in the setting of long-term secondary prevention is an intriguing hypothesis that remains unanswered.

Beyond clinical phenotype, genotype assessment to inform clinical decision-making for antiplatelet therapy continues to undergo clinical investigation. Two large randomized clinical trials have been recently completed on this subject and show conflicting results. POPular Genetics was a large randomized open-label trial that enrolled 2488 patients with STEMI undergoing primary PCI and assigned them in a 1:1 ratio to *CYP2C19*-based genetic testing–guided

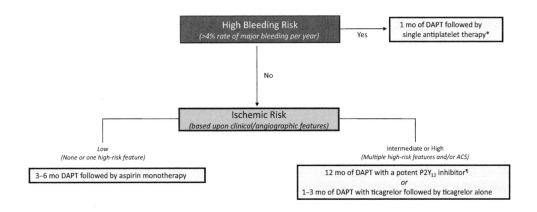

High bleeding risk is defined by the Academic Research Consortium (ARC-HBR) as a major bleeding rate of at least 4% at 1 y or intracranial hemorrhage risk of 1% at 1 y. Ischemic risk is categorized based upon clinical (diabetes mellitus requiring medication, peripheral arterial disease, acute coronary syndrome) and angiographic (multivessel PCI; stent length >60 mm; calcification requiring atherectomy) features associated with excess thrombosis. ACS – acute coronary syndrome. *HBR patients with concomitant atrial fibrillation receiving oral anticoagulation may be treated with clopidogrel alone and a direct oral anticoagulant. ¶ De-escalation from prasugrel or ticagrelor to clopidogrel may be considered based upon genetic or platelet function testing.

Fig. 2. Decision-making algorithm regarding DAPT in patients undergoing PCI. HBR is defined by Academic Research Council (ARC-HBR) as a bleeding risk of at least 4% at 1 year or intracranial hemorrhage risk of 1% at 1 year. Low ischemic risk includes Type A lesions and patients without multiple comorbidities. Intermediate/High ischemic risk includes patients who meet TWILIGHT trial inclusion criteria with or without ACS.

strategy (intervention) or standard treatment (either ticagrelor or prasugrel).[38] Patients with the loss of function alleles *CYP2C19* *2 and/or *3 received ticagrelor or prasugrel, whereas noncarriers of these mutations received clopidogrel. The genotype-guided strategy was noninferior for the primary composite outcome of net adverse clinical events (5.1% vs 5.9%, absolute difference, −0.7%, P<.001 for noninferiority) and superior for primary bleeding outcome (9.8% vs 12.5%, HR 0.78, P = .04) at 12 months' follow-up. TAILOR-PCI enrolled patients undergoing PCI for ACS or SIHD with planned 12 months of DAPT.[39] Similar to POPular genetics, the carriers in genotype-guided group received ticagrelor 90 mg twice daily, and noncarriers received clopidogrel 75 mg daily; however, an important difference from POPular genetics was that the control group received clopidogrel. Overall, the results of this trial were neutral as the primary end point occurred in 4.0% versus 5.9% (HR 0.66, P = .056) and TIMI major or minor bleeding occurred in 1.9% versus 1.6%; however, there was a 40% reduction in the cumulative primary endpoint events (P = .011), suggesting a signal of benefit for genotype-guided therapy. A very interesting post hoc analysis of this trial showed that 80% reduction in adverse events was observed during first 3 months of treatment in the genotype-guided group suggesting benefits in the early high-risk period after PCI.

SUMMARY

The decisions surrounding optimal duration and type of antiplatelet therapy should involve a careful assessment of individual patient ischemic and bleeding risk to optimize net-benefit. In patients with HBR, randomized evidence supports 1 month of DAPT followed by aspirin or $P2Y_{12}$ inhibitor.

In non-HBR patients who are at low ischemic risk, a short duration of DAPT followed by aspirin maybe reasonable. In non-HBR patients who are at intermediate to high ischemic risk (ACS presentation, multivessel disease, bifurcation disease, prior history of PCI, age >65, diabetes mellitus), 3 months of DAPT followed by ticagrelor monotherapy may be reasonable.

DISCLOSURE

Z.U.A. Asad has no financial disclosures. U. Baber discloses honoraria from Astra Zeneca, Boston Scientific, and Amgen.

REFERENCES

1. Alkhouli M, Alqahtani F, Kalra A, et al. Trends in characteristics and outcomes of patients undergoing coronary revascularization in the United States, 2003-2016. JAMA Netw Open 2020;3:e1921326.
2. Masoudi FA, Ponirakis A, de Lemos JA, et al. Trends in U.S. cardiovascular care: 2016 report from 4 ACC National Cardiovascular Data Registries. J Am Coll Cardiol 2017;69:1427–50.
3. Gruntzig A. Transluminal dilatation of coronary-artery stenosis. Lancet 1978;1:263.
4. Canfield J, Totary-Jain H. 40 years of percutaneous coronary intervention: history and future directions. J Pers Med 2018;8:33. Available at: https://www.ncbi.nlm.nih.gov/pmc/articles/PMC6313463/. Accessed April 26, 2020.
5. Amsterdam Ezra A, Wenger Nanette K, Brindis Ralph G, et al. 2014 AHA/ACC guideline for the management of patients with non–ST-elevation acute coronary syndromes. Circulation 2014;130:e344–426.
6. O'Gara PT, Kushner FG, Ascheim DD, et al. 2013 ACCF/AHA guideline for the management of ST-elevation myocardial infarction: a report of the American College of Cardiology Foundation/American Heart Association Task Force on Practice Guidelines. J Am Coll Cardiol 2013;61:e78–140.
7. Fihn Stephan D, Gardin Julius M, Abrams J, et al. 2012 ACCF/AHA/ACP/AATS/PCNA/SCAI/STS guideline for the diagnosis and management of patients with stable ischemic heart disease. Circulation 2012;126:e354–471.
8. 2011 ACCF/AHA/SCAI guideline for percutaneous coronary intervention | Circulation. Available at: https://www.ahajournals.org/doi/full/10.1161/cir.0b013e31823ba622. Accessed April 30, 2020.
9. 2015 ESC Guidelines for the management of acute coronary syndromes in patients presenting without persistent ST-segment elevation | European Heart Journal | Oxford Academic. Available at: https://academic-oup-com.webproxy2.ouhsc.edu/eurheartj/article/37/3/267/2466099. Accessed April 24, 2020.
10. Levine Glenn N, Bates Eric R, Bittl John A, et al. 2016 ACC/AHA guideline focused update on duration of dual antiplatelet therapy in patients with coronary artery disease: a report of the American College of Cardiology/American Heart Association Task Force on Clinical Practice Guidelines: an update of the 2011 ACCF/AHA/SCAI guideline for percutaneous coronary intervention, 2011 ACCF/AHA guideline for coronary artery bypass graft surgery, 2012 ACC/AHA/ACP/AATS/PCNA/SCAI/STS guideline for the diagnosis and management of patients with stable ischemic heart disease, 2013 ACCF/AHA guideline for the management of ST-elevation myocardial infarction, 2014 AHA/ACC

guideline for the management of patients with non–ST-elevation acute coronary syndromes, and 2014 ACC/AHA guideline on perioperative cardiovascular evaluation and management of patients undergoing noncardiac surgery. Circulation 2016; 134:e123–55.

11. Antithrombotic Trialists' (ATT) Collaboration, Baigent C, Blackwell L, et al. Aspirin in the primary and secondary prevention of vascular disease: collaborative meta-analysis of individual participant data from randomised trials. Lancet 2009; 373:1849–60.

12. Leon MB, Baim DS, Popma JJ, et al. A clinical trial comparing three antithrombotic-drug regimens after coronary-artery stenting. Stent Anticoagulation Restenosis Study Investigators. N Engl J Med 1998;339:1665–71.

13. Yusuf S, Zhao F, Mehta SR, et al. Effects of clopidogrel in addition to aspirin in patients with acute coronary syndromes without ST-segment elevation. N Engl J Med 2001;345:494–502.

14. Baber U, Dangas G, Chandrasekhar J, et al. Time-dependent associations between actionable bleeding, coronary thrombotic events, and mortality following percutaneous coronary intervention: results from the PARIS registry. JACC Cardiovasc Interv 2016;9:1349–57.

15. Mehran R, Baber U, Sharma SK, et al. Ticagrelor with or without aspirin in high-risk patients after PCI. N Engl J Med 2019;381:2032–42.

16. Hahn J-Y, Song YB, Oh J-H, et al. Effect of P2Y12 inhibitor monotherapy vs dual antiplatelet therapy on cardiovascular events in patients undergoing percutaneous coronary intervention: the SMART-CHOICE randomized clinical trial. JAMA 2019;321: 2428–37.

17. Vranckx P, Valgimigli M, Jüni P, et al. Ticagrelor plus aspirin for 1 month, followed by ticagrelor monotherapy for 23 months vs aspirin plus clopidogrel or ticagrelor for 12 months, followed by aspirin monotherapy for 12 months after implantation of a drug-eluting stent: a multicentre, open-label, randomised superiority trial. Lancet 2018; 392:940–9.

18. Watanabe H, Domei T, Morimoto T, et al. Effect of 1-month dual antiplatelet therapy followed by clopidogrel vs 12-month dual antiplatelet therapy on cardiovascular and bleeding events in patients receiving PCI. JAMA 2019;321:2414–27.

19. Yeh RW, Kereiakes DJ, Steg PG, et al. Lesion complexity and outcomes of extended dual antiplatelet therapy after percutaneous coronary intervention. J Am Coll Cardiol 2017;70:2213–23.

20. Stefanescu Schmidt Ada C, Kereiakes Dean J, Cutlip Donald E, et al. Myocardial infarction risk after discontinuation of thienopyridine therapy in the randomized DAPT study (dual antiplatelet therapy). Circulation 2017;135:1720–32.

21. Kedhi E, Fabris E, van der Ent M, et al. Six months versus 12 months dual antiplatelet therapy after drug-eluting stent implantation in ST-elevation myocardial infarction (DAPT-STEMI): randomised, multicentre, non-inferiority trial. BMJ 2018;363:k3793.

22. Baber U. Ticagrelor with aspirin or alone in high-risk patients After coronary intervention for acute coronary syndrome TWILIGHT-ACS. 24. Available at: https://professional.heart.org/idc/groups/ahamah-public/@wcm/@sop/@scon/documents/download-able/ucm_505186.pdf.

23. Giustino G, Harari R, Baber U, et al. Long-term safety and efficacy of new-generation drug-eluting stents in women with acute myocardial infarction. JAMA Cardiol 2017;2:855–62.

24. Baber U, Mehran R, Giustino G, et al. Coronary thrombosis and major bleeding after PCI with drug-eluting stents: risk scores from PARIS. J Am Coll Cardiol 2016;67:2224–34.

25. Angiolillo DJ, Baber U, Sartori S, et al. Ticagrelor with or without aspirin in high-risk patients with diabetes mellitus undergoing percutaneous coronary intervention. J Am Coll Cardiol 2020;75(19):2403–13.

26. Copeland-Halperin RS, Baber U, Aquino M, et al. Prevalence, correlates, and impact of coronary calcification on adverse events following PCI with newer-generation DES: findings from a large multiethnic registry. Catheter Cardiovasc Interv 2018;91:859–66.

27. Dangas G, Baber U, Sharma S, et al. Ticagrelor with aspirin or alone after complex PCI: the TWILIGHT-COMPLEX analysis. J Am Coll Cardiol 2020;75(19): 2414–24.

28. Giustino G, Chieffo A, Palmerini T, et al. Efficacy and safety of dual antiplatelet therapy after complex PCI. J Am Coll Cardiol 2016;68:1851–64.

29. Dangas GD, Claessen BE, Mehran R, et al. Development and validation of a stent thrombosis risk score in patients with acute coronary syndromes. JACC Cardiovasc Interv 2012;5:1097–105.

30. Armstrong PCJ, Leadbeater PD, Chan MV, et al. In the presence of strong P2Y12 receptor blockade, aspirin provides little additional inhibition of platelet aggregation. J Thromb Haemost 2011;9:552–61.

31. Baber U, Zafar MU, Dangas G, et al. Ticagrelor with or without aspirin after PCI: the TWILIGHT platelet substudy. J Am Coll Cardiol 2020;75: 578–86.

32. Franchi F, Rollini F, Aggarwal N, et al. Pharmacodynamic comparison of prasugrel versus ticagrelor in patients with type 2 diabetes mellitus and coronary artery disease: The OPTIMUS (Optimizing Antiplatelet Therapy in Diabetes Mellitus)-4 Study. Circulation 2016;134(11):780–92.

33. Urban P, Macaya C, Rupprecht HJ, et al. Randomized evaluation of anticoagulation versus

antiplatelet therapy after coronary stent implantation in high-risk patients: the multicenter aspirin and ticlopidine trial after intracoronary stenting (MATTIS). Circulation 1998;98:2126–32.

34. Kim B-K, Hong M-K, Shin D-H, et al. A new strategy for discontinuation of dual antiplatelet therapy: the RESET trial (REal safety and efficacy of 3-month dual antiplatelet therapy following endeavor zotarolimus-eluting stent implantation). J Am Coll Cardiol 2012;60:1340–8.

35. Feres F, Costa RA, Abizaid A, et al. Three vs twelve months of dual antiplatelet therapy after zotarolimus-eluting stents: the OPTIMIZE randomized trial. JAMA 2013;310:2510–22.

36. Bonaca MP, Bauersachs RM, Anand SS, et al. Rivaroxaban in peripheral artery disease after revascularization. N Engl J Med 2020;382:1994–2004.

37. Eikelboom JW, Connolly SJ, Bosch J, et al. Rivaroxaban with or without aspirin in stable cardiovascular disease. N Engl J Med 2017;377:1319–30.

38. Claassens DMF, Vos GJA, Bergmeijer TO, et al. A genotype-guided strategy for oral P2Y12 inhibitors in primary PCI. N Engl J Med 2019;381: 1621–31.

39. Tailored antiplatelet initiation to lessen outcomes due to decreased clopidogrel response after percutaneous coronary intervention. American College of Cardiology. Available at: http://%3a%2f%2fwww.acc.org%2flatest-in-cardiology%2fclinical-trials%2f2020%2f03%2f26%2f19%2f53%2ftailor-pci. Accessed May 9, 2020.

40. Windecker S, Latib A, Kedhi E, et al. Polymer-based or polymer-free stents in patients at high bleeding risk. N Engl J Med 2020;382:1208–18.

41. Ticagrelor with or without aspirin in acute coronary syndrome after PCI. American College of Cardiology. Available at: http://%3a%2f%2fwww.acc.org%2flatest-in-cardiology%2fclinical-trials%2f2020%2f03%2f27%2f22%2f47%2ftico. Accessed May 10, 2020.

Moving?

Make sure your subscription moves with you!

To notify us of your new address, find your **Clinics Account Number** (located on your mailing label above your name), and contact customer service at:

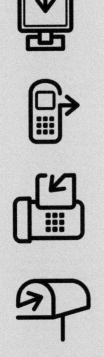

Email: journalscustomerservice-usa@elsevier.com

800-654-2452 (subscribers in the U.S. & Canada)
314-447-8871 (subscribers outside of the U.S. & Canada)

Fax number: 314-447-8029

Elsevier Health Sciences Division
Subscription Customer Service
3251 Riverport Lane
Maryland Heights, MO 63043

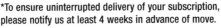
*To ensure uninterrupted delivery of your subscription, please notify us at least 4 weeks in advance of move.

ELSEVIER